Fit Foods and Fakeaways

Thorsons
An imprint of HarperCollins*Publishers*
1 London Bridge Street
London SE1 9GF

www.harpercollins.co.uk

HarperCollins*Publishers*
1st Floor, Watermarque Building,
Ringsend Road
Dublin 4, Ireland

First published by Thorsons 2021

10 9 8 7 6 5 4 3 2 1

Text © Courtney Black 2021
Photography © Anna Fowler 2021
Food photography © Sophie Fox 2021

Courtney Black asserts the moral right
to be identified as the author of this work

Contributing Writers: Jenny Francis and
Oliver Downey (food)
Stylist: Sarah-Rose Harrison
Hair: Jack Luckhurst
Make-up: Roqa Beauty
Food Stylist: Pippa Leon
Prop Stylist: Lauren Miller

A catalogue record of this book is
available from the British Library

ISBN 978-0-00-846854-5

Printed and bound by GPS

MIX
Paper from
responsible sources
FSC
www.fsc.org
FSC™ C007454

This book is produced from independently certified FSC™ paper
to ensure responsible forest management.

For more information visit: www.harpercollins.co.uk/green

COURTNEY BLACK

Thorsons

Fit Foods and Fakeaways
100 Healthy and Delicious Recipes

CONTENTS

Introduction

Hi!

When you mention food, especially in the fitness world, most people think of restriction: not eating certain foods, not consuming too many calories, not drinking alcohol . . .

So before we go any further, I want to tell you what this book is not.

This is not a diet plan.
This is not a weight-loss guide.
This is not a 'what-I-eat-in-a-day' book.
This is not a 'good' and 'bad' food manual.

To be clear: this book is not going to tell you what to eat and what not to eat. I'm not going to pretend that I can tell you the exact number of calories to consume to lose weight or the precise amount of protein to eat to gain muscle, as everyone needs different amounts, depending on many factors.

What I am going to do is use this book to arm you with all the information I can about food and nutrition with no quick fixes, no extreme calorie restrictions, no cutting out foods and no boring meals.

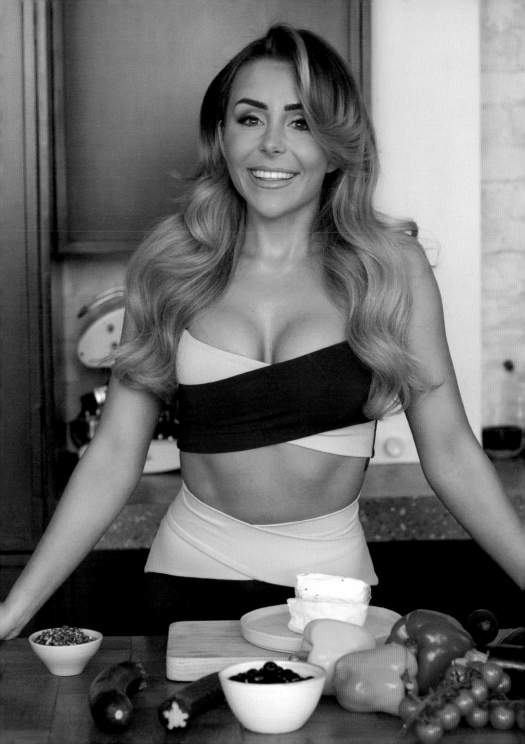

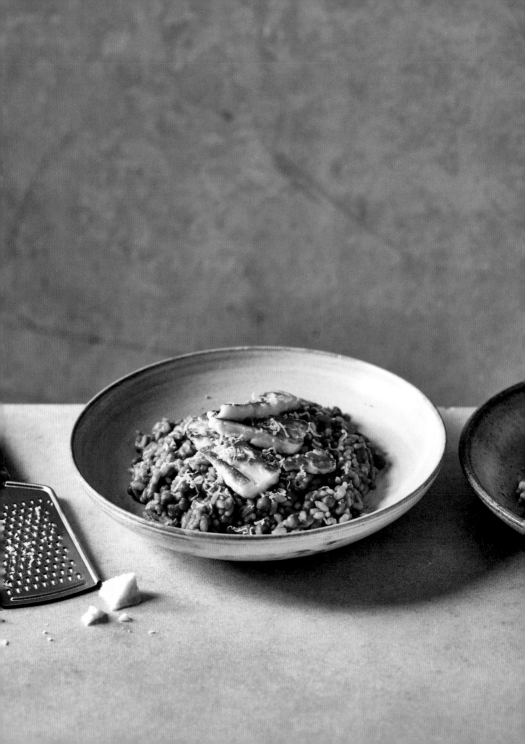

I'm going to tell you to ignore all the diet myths that you've been mis-sold in the past, so that you can make the food choices that are going to best benefit you going forward.

I am going to get you excited about food and cooking.

I am going to get you creative in the kitchen and banish any unhealthy relationships with food. I will not let you suffer in the way that I did.

If you're thinking, 'I don't want to know about food; I just want to know what to order at a restaurant that isn't going to make me gain weight', then you are the exact person who this book is aimed at.

I was you once. I didn't care about nutrition or macros or cooking for myself. I just wanted to know the 'cheats' to eating.

But there are no 'cheats' – only facts. And I promise that if you trust me to take you on this journey, by the time you reach the recipes, you'll be buzzing to get cooking.

So stop looking for quick fixes and remedies to help you lose weight or reach your goals. Let's focus on pleasure and living long and happy lives instead.

In my first book, *The Pocket PT*, I told you not to be too hard on yourself with fitness as everyone is a beginner once. And it's the same with food and diet. Whether you are confident in the kitchen or can barely make a piece of toast, with a better understanding of food and tons of delicious, easy-to-make recipes, you'll be eating your way to a fitter, healthier, happier you, and you'll love every mouthful.

Love,

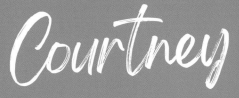

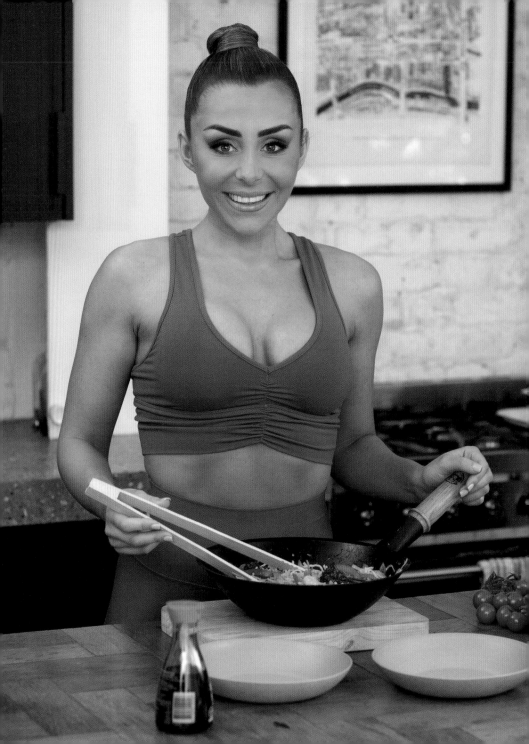

MY FOOD JOURNEY

Most of you who know me know about my personal journey with food, but I wanted to put a short version of it in this book because I think it is so important to remind you that no one is born with perfect food habits. We all have to go on a personal journey to find balance and, unfortunately, mine was quite extreme.

I have always been really open about how destructive my past eating and fitness habits were because it's important to me that you trust me and understand how long it has taken for me to get to where I am now.

I used to be a dancer. I competed in championships and I was in it because I just loved to dance. But competitions involve people looking at you and your body, so it makes you much more aware of what you look like in relation to other girls. I also had to wear tight-fitting outfits that showed a lot of skin, and I think it was a combination of all these things that led to me developing a really unhealthy relationship with food around the age of fifteen. I became obsessed with dieting, and never quite realised, until recently, how much I struggled with food.

It came from a destructive cycle of overthinking, obsessing about calories and restriction. Dancing made me compare myself to other girls, but then I found myself doing this outside of the dancing world, too.

I would watch music videos and the Victoria's Secret catwalk shows and vigorously exercise while doing so. It became an obsession – comparing and googling how to lose weight and get quick results.

I didn't know much about nutrition; I just thought I had to eat as little as possible. I followed the diet myths of not eating past 6pm and not eating carbs, both of which I can assure you are myths and don't work.

Of course, my weight dropped dramatically, but by this point, even though I didn't realise it, I was in the clutches of an eating disorder.

YOU CANNOT BE TRULY HAPPY LIVING A LIFE OF RESTRICTION IN FEAR OF FOOD.

I left dancing behind when I was sixteen, but needed something to fill the void, so I started exercising excessively instead.

I got my first job at seventeen, and spent every spare minute in the gym (there was one right under my office building). This is when the real problems started, as I never ate a proper meal and would train super early, before work, sometimes for two hours or more, and then again during my lunch break.

I had no energy, felt constantly faint during my gym sessions and made mistakes all the time at work because I couldn't concentrate. This led to me being frustrated on a regular basis. Imagine always being told you have made mistakes – it's so draining.

I also had absolutely no social life. I would turn down dinners, nights out and even work lunches because I was petrified of skipping a gym session and feared eating at a restaurant or going over my calorie allowance.

My body was craving nutrition and calories, but I saw food as the enemy, and so instead of giving my body what it wanted, I bought into all those awful 'fake foods', like 'zero-calorie soup', 'no-sugar chocolate' and 'diet bars'.

I would never allow myself chocolates or pasta and I repeatedly restricted myself, leading to a vicious cycle of disordered eating.

In the long run, I was doing my body so much harm physically, but there was also an emotional cost.

You cannot be truly happy living a life of restriction in fear of food.

I feel very lucky because things slowly changed for me when I decided to become a personal trainer. At the time, it was just part of my obsession, as I wanted to look my best and be the best version of myself.

But when I went on a course that forced me to learn about the body, nutrition and how it all works, I was made to break through the terrible mindset I'd been stuck in for years. I realised how little I knew in regards to nutrition and how much false information I had believed from the advertisements, shitty diet forums and even shittier magazines and newspapers that sell and promote these fad diets and diet myths.

The course made me face up to the facts, and the people I was surrounded by in the fitness environment helped me to understand that food was not the enemy.

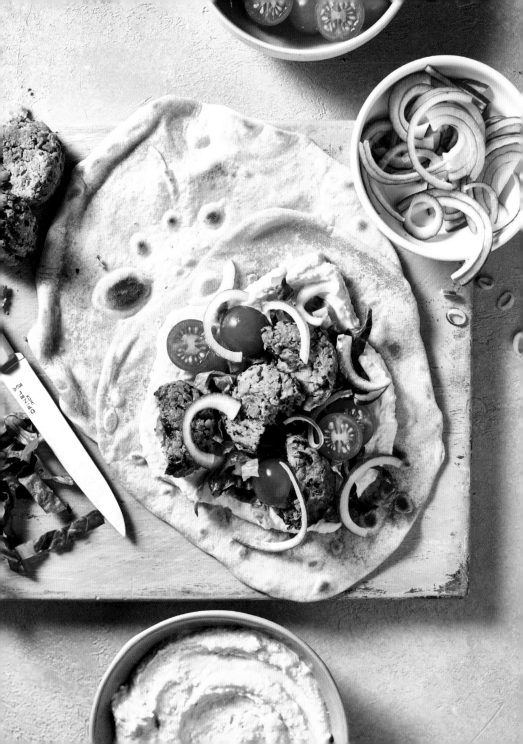

It was a very slow process, but my education on food and the body changed everything. It helped me stop undereating and – eventually – I was able to see how empowering a healthy diet could be, and how I didn't have to fear food any more.

I want to stress that this didn't happen overnight – it has taken me years to action this.

I can confidently say that I am now the happiest I have ever been and no longer recognise the girl I was – because I absolutely love food and cooking now. It's a huge part of my life and it's part of the reason that I wanted to write this book: I just want to share everything I've learned and all my favourite foods with you all.

Learning the basics of nutrition and home cooking is one of the most empowering things you can do. You can enjoy the most delicious food with no regret or guilt. You should never feel guilty about enjoying food . . . it's just food!

It's been a long journey, but one that, thank god, has led me to a more positive lifestyle.

I didn't want to listen to the experts; I thought I knew best. And I am asking you to not be this person. Trust in me as your trainer that your body needs food; food is neither 'good' nor 'bad' and you do not need to stop yourself eating at certain times to live a happy life.

WHY WE EAT

We eat to stay alive, yes, but if it was as simple as eating to live, we'd all just eat the same easy, healthy food every day. Food is so much more than that, which is why I chose to start this book with this little section, to remind us how what we eat impacts so much of who we are.

So what do we eat for?

Enjoyment

Food tastes good. It is such a huge part of our lives and our culture that we have to remember to enjoy every mouthful. If we forget to actually enjoy food, we are missing out on so much happiness.

So, before you go any further, just stop and read this bit again. Food is there to be enjoyed!

Energy

Our bodies can't function without energy and that energy comes from food. Calories are energy.

Whether it's walking to the shops, completing a workout, writing a presentation or even just breathing – everything we do takes up energy, and that's why it's so important that we eat enough food to power ourselves through every day.

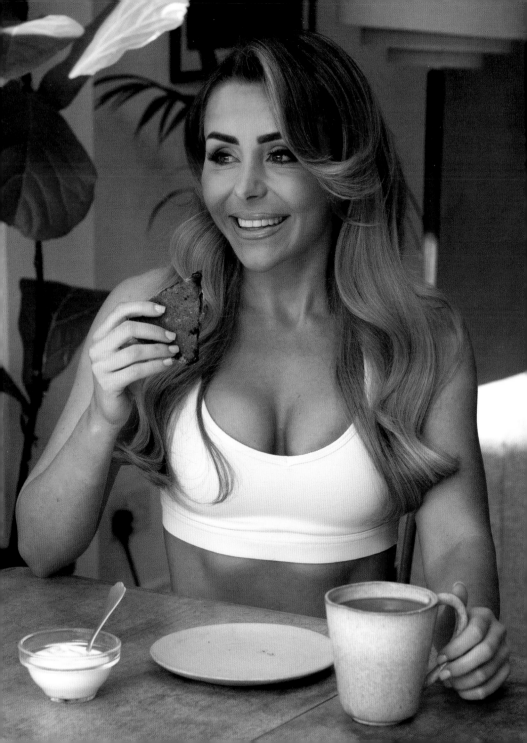

Your workout is such a small proportion of your day (let's just say around 3–4 per cent), so stop focusing on how many calories you burn in that time.

Mood

Just as our muscles need energy to move, our brains need it to function properly.

When you restrict the food and calories you eat, you are restricting how much energy your body has and therefore affecting your mood, too.

The word 'hangry' comes from a place of truth – we cannot focus or perform well when we do not eat enough.

We also aren't our happiest selves. I suffered with this for so many years, being rude to and distant from so many people, but it was simply down to undereating.

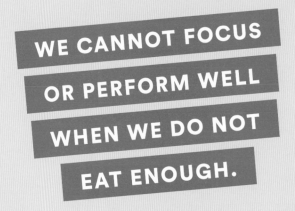

WE CANNOT FOCUS OR PERFORM WELL WHEN WE DO NOT EAT ENOUGH.

Sleep

Sleep is so incredibly important when it comes to our health, and what we eat – and how much – can contribute to how much sleep we get.

Both undereating and overeating can impact our ability to sleep well – it's a vicious cycle. If we sleep less, our body is low on energy, so we look to replace it with calories and food, which is why we are more likely to overeat when we are tired.

Health

If we don't eat, we can't survive. But the amount we eat (whether too much or too little) and what we eat (a varied, balanced diet or a restrictive, low-quality one) can impact our health in so many ways.

An unhealthy diet can lead to disease, obesity, infertility, mental-health problems and early death – so taking care of what we eat is hugely important.

GOOD MOOD FOOD

When we think about food, we usually think about it giving us energy and about how it impacts our physical bodies. But we often forget that food massively impacts our minds.

When I was undereating, I completely lost my personality. I was rude, irritable and couldn't take a joke. At times I was so exhausted I didn't have the energy to hold a conversation. (I know, can you imagine that?) Back then, I had no idea that my irritable mood was completely down to the fact that I was drastically undereating, and this was changing who I was.

I lost friends as a result. I had no social life, avoided birthday parties and social events and was terrified of being invited anywhere that involved eating.

Loads of studies have also found links between our stomachs and our brains. Continuous undereating or a very poor diet – only eating one type of food at every meal for example – mess with the body's regulation of insulin, causing inflammation and stress, which then transforms mood.

Eating healthy food helps the growth of 'good' bacteria, which then sends positive signals to your brain. Undereating, or a diet of junk and highly processed food, causes inflammation that stops the growth of these bacteria and prevents the positive signals from reaching your brain.

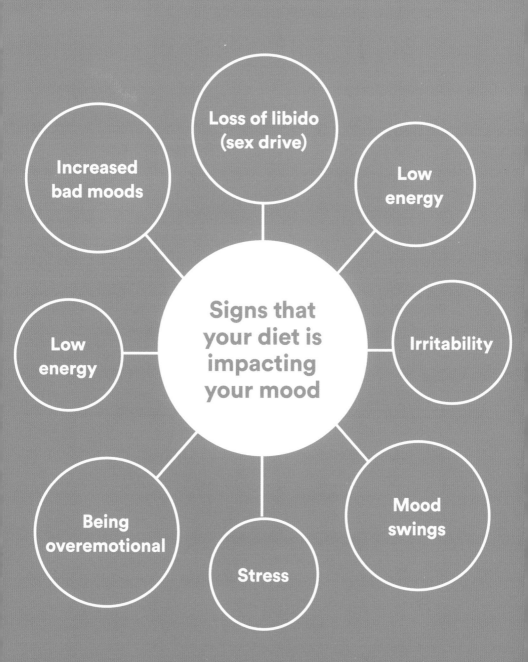

Loss of libido (sex drive)

Increased bad moods

Low energy

Low energy

Signs that your diet is impacting your mood

Irritability

Being overemotional

Stress

Mood swings

ARE YOU UNDER EATING?

When I was undereating, it was extreme and obsessive. But undereating isn't always as obvious as mine was.

When you start a fitness journey, the number of calories you burn in a day changes quite significantly. And as I touched on earlier, knowing exactly how many calories you burn is really difficult to measure – so it's not uncommon to massively underestimate how hard you worked during a training session, or to forget all those extra calories you burned while cleaning the house or popping to the shops.

When you train with me I never want you to starve yourself and I always recommend listening to your body. And that includes your hunger pangs. If you are feeling really hungry – eat something nutritious. Not only will this help feed your body when it needs it, it will also mean you can get on with your day without constantly thinking about food!

I just want to point out the obvious here – there is a big difference between listening to your body at 4pm and going to get a healthy snack and listening to your body at 11pm and going to get a family-size bar of chocolate.

But the point is that if you are exercising regularly, you need to fuel your body to be able to keep up your motivation, energy and mood.

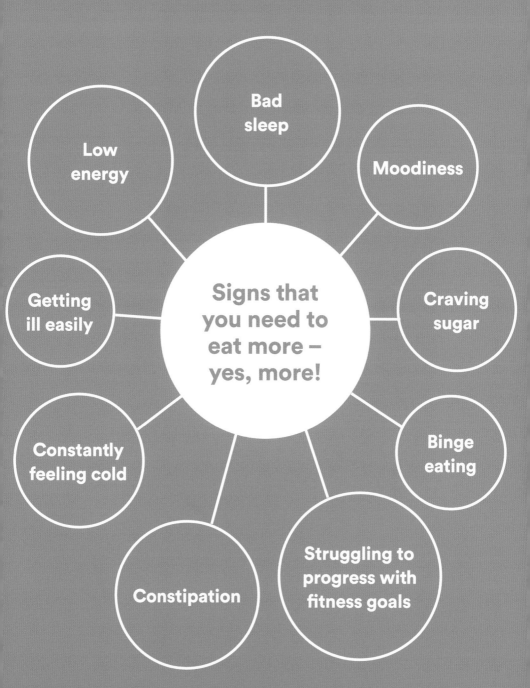

BINGE EATING

When we exercise regularly and take care of our diets by avoiding processed foods and making sure we eat a variety of nutrients, there are sometimes days – or whole weekends – when all our healthy intentions go out of the window and we decide to allow ourselves to eat and drink whatever we want.

First of all: this is normal. We all have lives outside of our workouts and that means social events, meals out and holidays – all the good stuff. And we've all been there when we've had a weekend binge and woken up on Monday feeling a little worse for wear because of a few days on a poor- quality diet.

This is absolutely fine. Until you feel guilty about it.

People message me all the time saying, 'I completely let myself go over the weekend and ruined my diet – what do I do?'

There is only one response and that is: relax and move on. The minute you start to punish yourself for having a good time or enjoying food is the minute you set yourself up for failure.

Food should never be associated with guilt, so instead, enjoy the memories of that amazing weekend you just had and use it to motivate yourself to enjoy the benefits of eating a more balanced diet over the next few days.

What you absolutely should not do is starve yourself for the next week 'to make up for it'. Or jump on a running machine and punish yourself with two hours of cardio to try to 'burn it all off'. This is really negative behaviour, and you are worth so much more than that.

So if you have had a few days of overeating, the best thing to do is just crack on with your normal, healthy routine.

I just want to say here that there is a big difference between occasional binge eating and the ongoing, extreme binge eating associated with disorders. In the case of the latter, you should seek immediate professional help, but if you detect a regular pattern to your bingeing – say, only at weekends – you should check in with yourself to adjust the things that might be contributing:

- Have you been restricting yourself with too few calories all week?
- Have you been overexercising without fuelling your body?
- Have you been forgetting to prioritise sleep?
- Are you going through a highly stressful or emotional time in your life?

I understand you might have a busy job and you may feel stressed, but why resort to food and alcohol? We shouldn't feel the need to go crazy on weekends; they are just like any other day. Saving yourself for the weekend often leads to weekend bingeing and, most of the time, not even enjoying it as much as you would if you just had that glass of wine when you wanted it most on a Tuesday night.

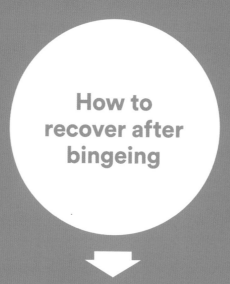

How to recover after bingeing

Get back to your eating plan or healthy recipes.

Get back to your exercise routine.

Don't obsess over it once it's happened: acknowledge the reasons why and learn from it.

Relax and move on.

Don't punish yourself for days after.

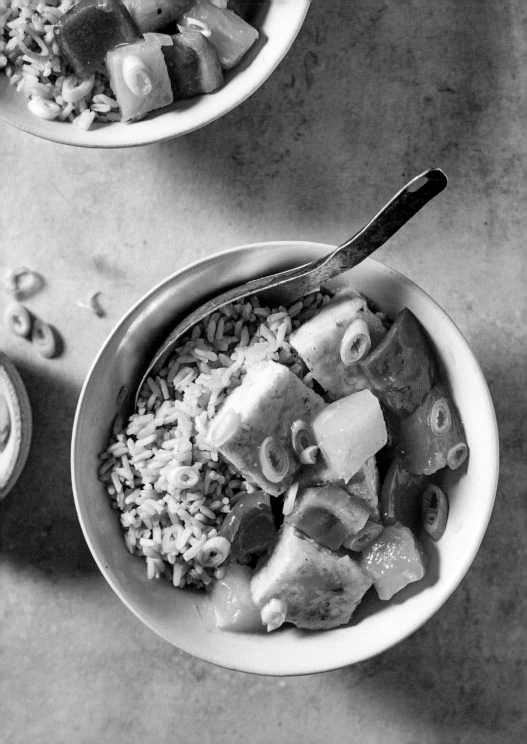

NUTRITION – THE BASICS

I wouldn't take you into a gym for the first time and just say 'Exercise!' But when it comes to nutrition, we are often left to our own devices.

We walk into a supermarket wanting to make healthy choices, but feel overwhelmed and totally lost as to what to put in our baskets.

Nutrition is very complex and scientific, but I want to simplify it here to make things easier to understand when it comes to everyday eating because I think that learning the basics is one of the most empowering things you can do.

Know your macros

I'm sure you've heard the word 'macros' bandied about in the fitness world when it comes to diet. But unlike a lot of buzzwords around food, this is one that's actually worth knowing about. It's short for macronutrients and is basically a way of putting all the main foods we eat into three categories:

- Proteins
- Fats
- Carbohydrates

Macronutrients provide us with two things: energy and substance for growth and maintenance.

They are divided up like this because each of the three types is used by the body in a slightly different way. And we need all three – yes, all three – for optimal health. That's why diets that cut out an entire macro food group are never going to end well.

- **Proteins** are basically what build the body. They make up everything from your hair and nails to your bones and muscles, making them work the way they should.
- **Fats** provide the body with energy and help to protect your organs and keep your body warm. They also make it possible for the body to absorb some key nutrients and produce hormones.
- **Carbohydrates** are our energy source. The body loves them and converts them to glucose to power us through the day. We can also store carbs for future energy, while the fibre in wholefood carbs is essential for good digestive health.

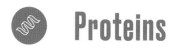

Proteins

Know your proteins

Protein can be found in some of my favourite foods. It's not all chicken and egg whites — meat, fish, dairy and plant-based foods are all great, high-quality sources of protein.

A lot of people, especially those who are very active, struggle to meet their protein goals, particularly those who are new to vegetarian and vegan diets. It's really important to know your protein sources though, so that you can easily include them in your daily meals and enjoy a variety of different versions of this macronutrient.

Meat/dairy protein sources

Cheese

Fish

Meat
(poultry, beef, pork)

Yogurt

Milk

Eggs

Shellfish

Vegetable proteins

Tofu

Lentils

Nuts

Spinach

Peas

Chia seeds

Broccoli

Buckwheat

Beans

Chickpeas

Nut butter

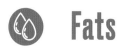

Fats

Know your fats

Fats have been demonised for years in the diet industry, but so many dietary fats are really, really good for us.

As I've said, I don't label foods as 'good' and 'bad' because I really believe that there is a place for every food in a balanced diet and I don't like to make any food the enemy, but to give you a bit of guidance on fats, I want to list those that I include most in my weekly diet.

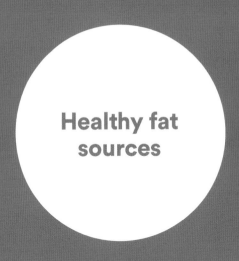

Healthy fat sources

Avocado

Nuts

Olives

Cheese

Nut butters

Tofu

Eggs

Dark chocolate

Sundried tomatoes

Olive oil

Salmon

Oily fish

Red meat

Yoghurts

Seeds

Chia seeds

Single cream

Crème fraîche

Coconut oil

Carbs

Know your carbs

Let's talk carbs. If you are a similar age to me, we have grown up being taught that carbs equals putting on weight. Carbs are 'the enemy', and so carbs are 'bad'.

But, as I've said, no food group is all bad and that couldn't be more true than it is of carbs.

I eat carbs every day and I absolutely love them. They taste great, give me energy and do not make me put on a stone in weight the minute I eat them.

Part of the reason there is so much confusion and demonising of carbohydrates is that people don't often know that there are different types of carbs and they do different things when we eat them.

To fully understand this food group, and to get rid of all of these myths surrounding it, we have to make an effort to learn the basics about carbohydrates so we can decide how to include them in our diets.

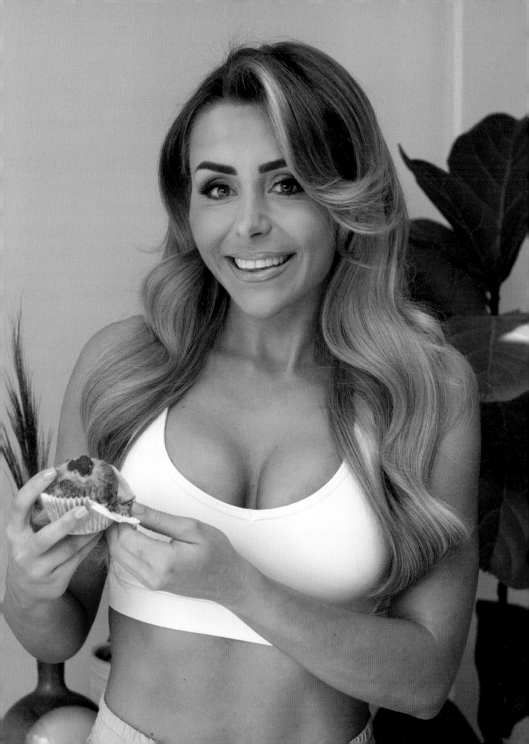

There are two kinds of carbohydrates: whole and refined.

- **Whole carbs** are unprocessed, natural and contain natural fibre.
- **Refined carbs** have been processed and the natural fibre is removed or changed as a result.

These two different types have very different nutritional qualities and so one type is a lot healthier than the other.

Refined carbs cause spikes in our blood-sugar levels, which can lead to a crash afterwards that triggers hunger and food cravings. They also lack essential nutrients, and the majority contain added sugar.

Lots of studies have shown that diets very high in refined carbs are linked with health conditions such as obesity and type 2 diabetes.

Having said all that, as with everything I say about diets, I'm not telling you that you should never eat refined carbs or that you should demonise them. I am simply arming you with the basic knowledge around food groups, so that you can choose which to include more or less of in your own personal diet.

Examples of whole carbs

Vegetables
Quinoa
Barley
Legumes
Potatoes
Wholegrains
Wholewheat pasta
Brown rice
Beans
Oats
Sweet potatoes
Wholegrain cereal
Wholemeal bread
Fruit

Examples of refined carbs

White bread
White pasta
White rice
Pastries
Chocolate and sweets
Non-diet fizzy drinks
Biscuits
Crisps
Pasteurised fruit juice
Sweets
Cakes

Calories

OK, guys. It's the big one: calories.

Calories are a really simple concept when it comes to food and diet – but for some reason they have been made so confusing.

It might surprise you to hear that I'm going to cover the topic of calories in just a couple of pages because I really don't think it takes any more than that for you to understand everything you need to know.

The amount of energy in the food or drink we consume is measured in calories.

Our bodies need to burn calories every second of the day, whether we are moving around, concentrating hard or even sleeping. So we need to nourish and care for our bodies by feeding them calories when needed.

When we consume more calories than we use up, our bodies store the excess energy as body fat. If we consume fewer calories than we use up, our bodies use the stored energy for fuel.

And it is as simple as that. I promise you.

So many people ask me what foods they should eat or avoid in order to lose weight. But it doesn't matter if you eat this or that at this or that time or drink this drink with that meal. The thing that makes you gain weight is simply consuming more calories than you use. It's so easy to overthink weight gain, but this really is all you need to know.

Using the example that you are burning 2,000 calories a day:

Your body burns 2,000 calories

+

you eat 2,000 calories

=

you maintain your body weight

Your body burns 2,000 calories

+

you eat 2,500 calories

=

you gain weight

Your body burns 2,000 calories

+

you eat 1,500 calories

=

you lose weight

YOUR PERSONAL DIET

So here is where some people would normally go on for pages, telling you exactly what a 'healthy macro split' looks like and precisely how many calories you should consume to lose or maintain weight. I'm going to do the total opposite.

When I decided to write a recipe book that was all about food and nutrition, I worried that people would think it was a weight-loss plan promising to tell them exactly what to eat in order to achieve their bodyweight goals. And the reason why I worried was because I know that is just not possible.

To me, this is the most important section in this book – and I wish I could write some magic words and recipes and tell you that 'If you eat these exact foods in these exact proportions, you will succeed in your body goals'. But the truth is that without knowing how much you are training, your daily movement, your age, your body shape, sleep patterns and your aims I can't begin to suggest a calorie goal for you.

Calorie intake and your macronutrient ratio are personalised to you and your goals.

That is why I want to keep coming back to the same message throughout this book, and that is: you will only find long-term success in your diet if you do you.

Only you know your weekly movement, your sleep patterns, the amount you fidget, the type of training you do and the type of foods you prefer eating.

No one else can ever work this out for you, so it would be one big, fat lie to put that information in this book, promising a one-size-fits-all solution.

If you really struggle to even come close to being able to estimate what your personal calorie intake should be to achieve your goals, there are loads of calorie calculators online that can help. Or you can download my Courtney Black app and enter in all your information to get a really good starting point.

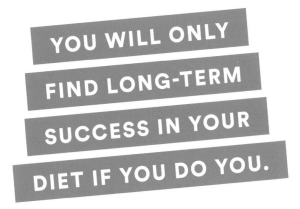

YOU WILL ONLY FIND LONG-TERM SUCCESS IN YOUR DIET IF YOU DO YOU.

BUSTING DIET MYTHS

'I read that if you eat food after 8pm it doubles the calories.'

'I saw on Instagram that if you have these diet shakes instead of breakfast you'll lose weight.'

'My friend said she lost weight because she stopped eating carbs.'

I'd need another ten books to be able to list all of the ridiculous things I've been told about diets and weight loss. And I'd need another ten to be able to go through them all and tell you why they are a load of rubbish.

But I wanted to include some of them in this book in order to help you understand how simple dieting is so that you can recognise nonsense diet information when you see it – and ignore it.

Here are some of the most common diet myths I have come across:

Myth: eating late at night = more calories

One of the biggest diet myths out there is that eating after a certain time of the day means you are more likely to put on body weight. This is incorrect and, to be honest, it makes me laugh because it's so ridiculous.

A 490-calorie meal at 5pm is still the same 490-calorie meal at 8pm, 9pm or even later. And a tub of Ben & Jerry's ice cream doesn't suddenly contain quadruple the calories at night. What makes you gain weight is if you have eaten 2,000 calories that day and then add another 490 at 9pm, when you have burned 2,000 calories already and are unlikely to burn many more before bed.

We need to get out of the mindset that we cannot eat after a certain time at night because it feeds into negative thought patterns and over-obsession about food.

Myth: eating carbs makes you gain weight

Carbs have been demonised in the diet and fitness world for years. As we've seen, refined carbs are much less nutritionally healthy for us than whole carbs, but when it comes to weight gain, the truth is, it doesn't matter which carbs – or how many of them – you choose to eat, as long as the number of calories you consume on any given day doesn't outweigh what you use.

Myth: one unhealthy meal cancels out everything else

This is a big one – and once you stop telling yourself this, it could transform your mindset when it comes to food.

Achieving our weight goals isn't about avoiding high-calorie foods for every meal or snack. If we allow ourselves to enjoy a takeaway burger or a chocolate brownie, that doesn't mean we have 'failed' that day.

Yes, we might have consumed more calories than we wanted to in one sitting, and we might not have given ourselves the best nutrition in the world, but it's just one meal in an entire day's worth of eating.

Instead of telling yourself that 'I've eaten one unhealthy thing, so I might as well consume all the other unhealthy things in the house because I've ruined my healthy eating plans for the day', take a second to remind yourself that it just isn't true.

If you have a burger for lunch, but then a home-cooked chicken breast and some veg for dinner, that is going to be much healthier for you than having a burger for lunch, then ordering fish and chips for dinner, eating a sharing-size bar of chocolate and finishing off the day with a tub of ice cream.

Balance out your healthy choices with your unhealthy choices and you'll set yourself up for long-term success.

Myth: fasting makes you lose weight quicker

Fasting is a big one at the moment. There is a lot of chat about not eating before 12pm to lose weight or going on extremely low-calorie diets for five days of the week to 'fast track' your weight loss.

The first thing I want to say here is that there is nothing wrong with fasting and there is nothing wrong with choosing to eat your meals at certain times of the day. But neither of these makes you lose weight any quicker or more effectively than any other diet you choose to follow.

It all comes down to the same thing, and that's the number of calories you have consumed on any given day versus how many you have burned. And that's the same whether you have skipped breakfast or not.

Myth: meal-replacement shakes are the secret to weight loss

If you ever see a diet product that claims to help you lose weight quicker than eating real food, ignore it – it is a lie. There are no quick fixes when it comes to losing weight.

Just like any other food, meal-replacement shakes don't make you miraculously start burning fat and they don't make you lose weight any quicker than eating a meal containing the exact same number of calories.

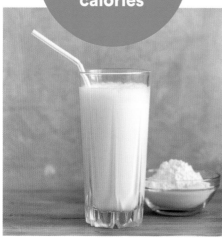

Meal replacement shake 400 calories

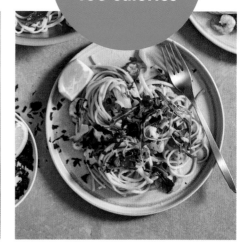

Courtney Black recipe 400 calories

Which would you prefer?

? Myth busting: a final word

This book is my way of saying – let's stop looking for quick fixes and diet 'cheats' and start looking for something you can stick to long term.

If I can help you to create a healthier and happier lifestyle by understanding food and nutrition, I hope I can also help you to understand that you don't have to waste money on 'fat-burning' products or quick-fix meal replacements.

Instead, you can focus on your own nutrition and energy expenditure and forget about everyone else's. This is how you are going to learn to enjoy food and love the feeling you get when you find that healthy balance.

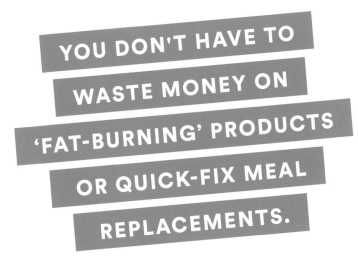

YOU DON'T HAVE TO WASTE MONEY ON 'FAT-BURNING' PRODUCTS OR QUICK-FIX MEAL REPLACEMENTS.

LEARNING FROM PREVIOUS MISTAKES

As soon as you get into the mindset of 'success' and 'failure', you are more likely to see an unhealthy choice as negative and feel bad about it. So it's really important when starting a new journey to healthy habits to know that you cannot fail.

I went through years of making bad choices with my diet before I learned where I'd been going wrong. It doesn't matter what your previous mistakes have been with food – and mine really were epic – as long as you learn from them.

So it might be that you had a huge binge for a whole weekend and overate processed foods. Of course, this isn't healthy, but you can learn from it. How did you feel afterwards? Lacking energy? Poor sleep? Didn't want to train?

And what made you do it? Undereating the week before? Punishing yourself for eating one unhealthy thing? Overtraining?

Basically, don't beat yourself up about your food choices. You can learn so much from the mistakes you make with your diet and use them to pick yourself up and become healthier and more knowledgeable going forwards.

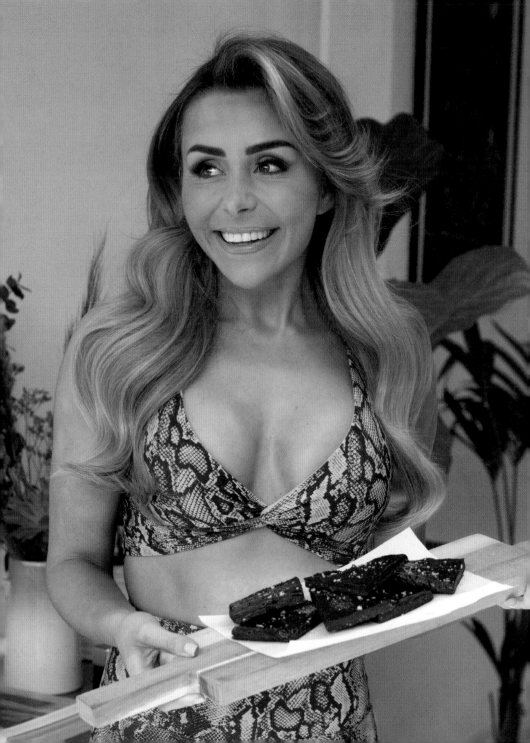

SETTING CALORIE TARGETS TOO LOW

So I've given you my take on calories and explained the importance of fuelling your body and now I just want to bring the two together because this is where so many people go wrong when they change their diets.

They decide they want to be in a calorie deficit – great. But instead of setting a target that gives them enough fuel to power them through their workouts and the energy to go to work or do the school run, they massively cut their calories so low that they can't possibly maintain eating so little. This is the easiest way to ruin any healthy-eating plans you had, along with your chances of reaching your goals.

So I just want to say it one more time: you don't need to cut your calorie intake down to a crazy low of, say, 800 calories a day to lose weight. It's unsustainable, it's unhealthy and it's unlikely that you will be able to keep up any sort of exercise routine.

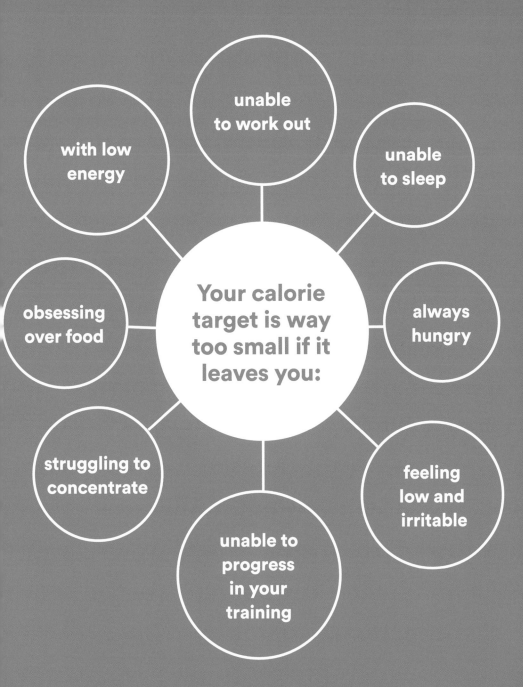

FALLING IN LOVE WITH HOME COOKING

I used to want to eat out all the time because the food I was making myself at home was bland and boring. I didn't realise that what I was cooking made me miserable because I was adding absolutely no flavour to it. I genuinely believed that if it tasted good, it had to be unhealthy and loaded with unnecessary calories. But the minute I started to learn about food and nutrition and how to cook for myself, I began to understand that I could be healthier and stop craving takeaways or going out for dinner all the time.

Flavour comes from all sorts of places and you can transform a meal into exactly what you fancy with just a few ingredients. I laugh when my friends say 'Courtney always has stuff to rustle up a meal' – but it's true. My cupboards are always stocked with basic ingredients, so that I can make a banging curry, stir-fry or bake at a moment's notice.

Now I look forward to cooking my own food even more than I do going out to eat because I've learned how to make my meals taste amazing and I know exactly what goes into them. Just learning simple cooking basics has transformed my life, my health and saved me loads of money. And I want to give you that same confidence in the kitchen so that you can create your favourite foods in a healthy way, too.

Benefits of cooking from scratch

Who doesn't love the novelty of having someone else cook for them? But when you are trying to be healthier or attempting to achieve a calorie deficit, eating out can be confusing. And when it comes to ready meals, yes, they are crazy convenient, but you need to look at the packet to see what ingredients they contain – if there is a long list of weird words you cannot even pronounce, that's when you know it's a no-go.

So sure, while these things can definitely have a place in your lifestyle from time to time, being able to cook from scratch as much as possible is what's really going to transform your ability to control what you eat.

Home cooking is amazing because:

1. You control what goes into food.
Cooking for yourself means you can choose things like how much salt to add, brown or white rice, adding sugar (or not). And it also means you know that there are no weird chemical preservatives involved.

2. You learn more about food.
When I started cooking, I really started to learn more about food – seeing what flavours go together, how different foods are cooked, incorporating a mix of different macros and understanding portion control were all part of my cooking journey. It just opens your mind to all the ways to make food healthier and more enjoyable to eat.

3. You can get creative with food.

You might learn how to make ten recipes, but that can become thirty when you start to improvise in the kitchen and come up with your own yummy recipes. Try simple substitutions of different ingredients to put a new twist on recipes you already know.

4. You enjoy the food more.

There is nothing more satisfying than eating a really delicious meal that you have made yourself. I always feel so proud when I make something I've never made before and it's just so empowering to know that I can cook nutritious food for myself without having to rely on a ready meal or someone else doing it for me.

Making my recipes work for you

I can't wait for you to try the recipes in this book. I have put so much effort into every single one of them and they are some of my favourite meals that I have created during my home-cooking journey.

While I have chosen my favourite ingredients for each meal, it's really important for you to use them in a way that makes them best suit you. For example, I love the Cheat's Chicken Katsu Curry (see page 90), but chicken might be your least favourite meat, or maybe you are a vegetarian. That doesn't mean you can't love this recipe though; just swap out the chicken for prawns or your favourite vegetable and make it your own.

That's what is so exciting about food – one recipe can be changed in endless different ways to make it something that is delicious to you.

Every recipe in this book is designed to fit into a healthy diet that will help you achieve your own personal goals, so adapting them with foods that suit you and your diet needs is absolutely something I encourage you to do.

Simple swaps

meat	➜	**fish or vegetables**
dairy sauces like cream and crème fraîche	➜	**coconut milk or yoghurt**
rice or pasta	➜	**baked potato**
eggs	➜	**tofu**
olive oil	➜	**coconut oil**
white potato	➜	**sweet potato**

Why I love fakeaways

I get messages from thousands of people every day asking for diet advice, and one thing that comes up again and again is a love of takeaways. Whether it's pizza, fish and chips or a Chinese, takeaways are something that so many people have grown to love, but loads of them tell me they don't feel they can fit them into their fitness goals.

Firstly, you can still enjoy takeaways – in moderation, of course. As I gained more knowledge about nutrition I realised two things:

    1. A lot of takeaways are really well-balanced meals – it's just the way they are cooked that makes them unhealthy.

    2. They are also some of the easiest meals to make at home – only with fewer calories and without the ultra-processed ingredients found in the ones you order to your door.

    I also realised that cooking them from scratch was so much cheaper than ordering them in – but that was just a bonus.

    I loved coming up with ways to recreate takeaways at home, and they are always so popular on my social media that I couldn't resist coming up with some more and sharing them with you here as part of this recipe book.

    I honestly love all the recipes in this book, but my absolute favourites are the Prawn Tacos (see page 112), Spaghetti Bolognese (see page 118) and the Blueberry Scones (see page 204). And I can't wait to hear which ones you love best! Now, let's get cooking . . .

Takeaway vs Fakeaway

Fakeaway Five Girls Burger:

Carbs 28.6g

Calories 495

Fat 40.1g

Protein 63.5g

Takeaway Double Cheese Burger:

Carbs 40

Calories 968

Fat 69g

Protein 52g

(Source myfitnesspal)

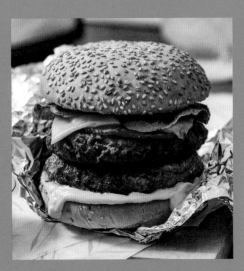 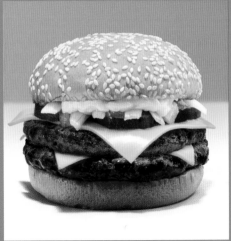

Which would you prefer?

BREAKFAST

Carbs 41g

Calories 275

Fat 5.2g

Protein 15g

Baked Berry Oats

A lovely way to begin your day. The natural sweetness of the syrup and fruit makes this dish feel like a big hug first thing in the morning.

SERVES 4

1 scoop vanilla protein powder
½ tsp baking powder
1 free-range egg, beaten
280ml skimmed milk
1 tbsp maple syrup
150g rolled oats
1 tsp chia seeds
1 level tsp ground cinnamon
400g frozen mixed berries
1 tbsp fresh mint leaves, to serve

1. Preheat the oven to 200°C/400°F/Gas 6.
2. Mix the protein powder, baking powder, egg, milk and maple syrup in a bowl.
3. Mix together the oats, chia seeds and cinnamon.
4. Place half of the berries in the bottom of a baking dish and sprinkle over half of the oats. Pour half the milk mixture over the top, then add the rest of the oats, the remaining milk mixture and the rest of the berries on top.
5. Bake in the oven for 25 minutes until the milk has been absorbed and it has begun to turn golden.
6. Serve with the fresh mint leaves sprinkled over.

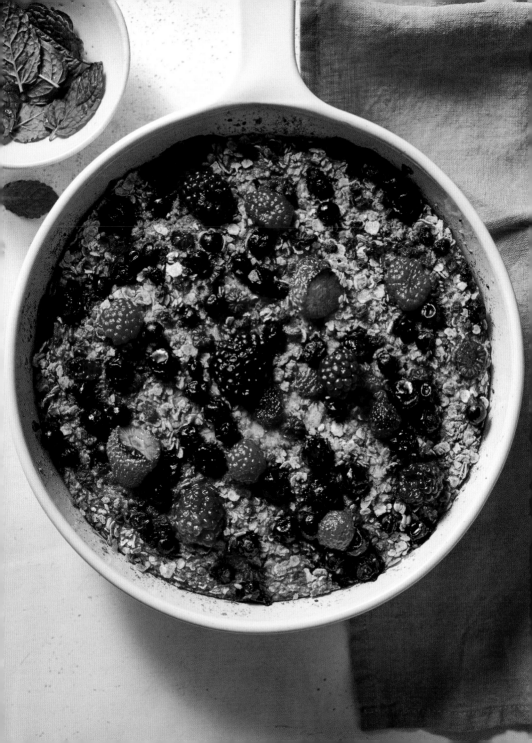

Carbs 50.5g

Calories 321

Fat 5.3g

Protein 18.3g

Vegan Chocolate Orange Overnight Oats

These quick overnight oat pots are packed with protein, with the perfect amount of sweetness from the orange.

SERVES 2

80g rolled oats

1 scoop chocolate protein powder (vegan)

1 large orange, zest and flesh cut into segments

200ml unsweetened almond milk

1 tbsp maple syrup

1 tbsp unsweetened cacao nibs

1. In a glass jar, bowl or container, mix together the oats, protein powder and orange zest until well combined.
2. Pour in the almond milk and maple syrup and stir well.
3. Pop in the fridge overnight and, when you are ready to serve, top with the cacao nibs and orange segments.

Carbs 33.1g

Calories 398

Fat 11.3g

Protein 40.1g

Croque Monsieur

This famous Parisian dish is made with fat-free quark, which is high in protein. Use whichever bread you prefer, but I love crusty white bread.

SERVES 2

1 tbsp plain quark

30g reduced-fat Cheddar, grated

30g reduced-fat mozzarella, grated

1 tsp Dijon mustard

4 slices crusty white bread

4 slices thick, lean ham

Low-calorie cooking spray

Salad leaves, to serve

1. Preheat the grill to medium.
2. In a small bowl, mix together the quark, two-thirds of the cheeses and the Dijon mustard.
3. Divide the mixture between two slices of bread and top with the ham, followed by the remaining slices of bread.
4. Heat a frying pan over a medium heat and spray the top of the bread with the low-calorie cooking spray. Place the sandwiches in the pan, oiled side down, and fry for 2–3 minutes until golden.
5. While the bottoms cook, spray the sides facing up with the cooking spray, then flip and fry until golden.
6. Once both sides are crisp and golden, place the sandwiches on a baking tray and top with the remaining cheese. Pop under the preheated grill for 2–3 minutes until the cheese has melted. Serve with some fresh salad leaves.

Carbs 55g

Calories 425

Fat 8g

Protein 34g

Courtney's Famously Fluffy Protein Pancakes

These fluffy protein pancakes are bursting with protein and taste just like the real American version.

SERVES 1
1 scoop vanilla protein powder
1 banana
1 free-range egg
20g oats
½ tbsp baking powder
Dash of milk (almond or oat)
Low-calorie cooking spray

TO SERVE
50g blueberries
1 tsp honey

1. Blend all the ingredients (except the cooking spray and serving ingredients) in a food processor. The mixture should be quite thick and not runny.
2. Heat your pan over a medium heat, so the pancakes cook slower and don't burn.
3. Spray your pan with the cooking spray ready for cooking.
4. Add a spoonful or ladleful of mixture to the pan. The mix should make around six pancakes, so pour slowly and eyeball how big they need to be.
5. Cook for about 2 minutes on each side. Serve with the blueberries and honey.

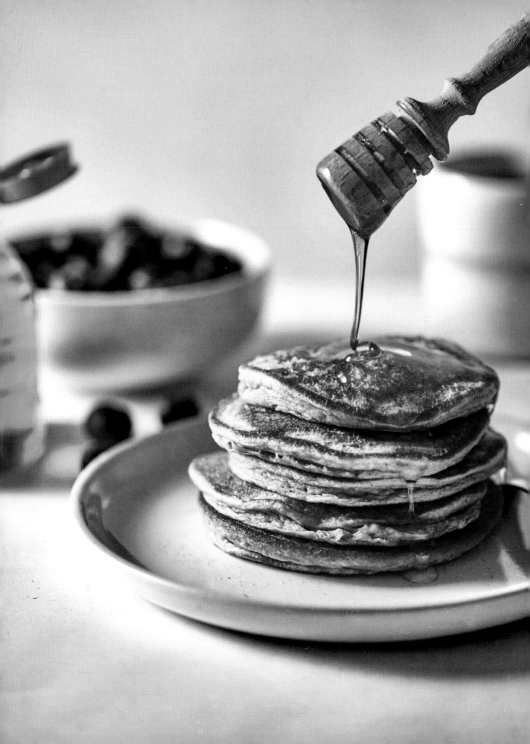

Carbs 31g	
Calories 330	
Fat 14g	
Protein 24g	

Eggs Benedict

This is such a classic breakfast, we just had to include it. Hollandaise sauce usually calls for enormous amounts of butter, but we've swapped the butter for yoghurt here to make a low-calorie, high-protein version. There are quite a few steps to this recipe, but the end result is totally worth it!

SERVES 2
2 large free-range eggs
2 English breakfast muffins
150g baby spinach
2 slices honey-roast smoked ham (we prefer thick-sliced, but use whichever you can find)
¼ tsp cayenne pepper

FOR THE HOLLANDAISE SAUCE
2 free-range egg yolks
60g fat-free yoghurt
1 tsp white wine vinegar
½ tsp Dijon mustard (optional)

1. To make the hollandaise sauce, fill a saucepan with a couple of centimetres of water and place a heatproof glass bowl over it, ensuring that it doesn't touch the water (if it does, just get rid of some of the water). The steam from the water in the pan will heat the glass bowl and cook the egg yolk, but if the water is touching the bottom of the glass dish, it will be too hot, and the egg will scramble instead. Once you have checked that the level is right, remove the bowl and place the saucepan over a medium heat until the water is steaming, but not boiling.
2. In the glass bowl, whisk together the egg yolks and the yoghurt and place over the saucepan.
3. Keep whisking over the heat until the mixture thickens. This can take anywhere from 10 to 15 minutes. If the water begins to boil, reduce the heat.
4. Once the sauce has thickened, remove the bowl from the heat, whisk in the white wine vinegar and Dijon, if using, then set aside while you make the poached eggs. (It can always be reheated if it gets cold.)
5. Half fill another saucepan with water, bring to the boil and, once boiling, swirl it with the end of a wooden spoon to create a small whirlpool.
6. Crack the eggs in, turn the heat off and leave to cook for 3–4 minutes. As the eggs are cooking, pop a colander on top of the pan and steam the spinach until wilted.

7. Meanwhile, toast the muffins.
8. To check if the eggs are cooked, lift one out of the water with a slotted spoon and if the whites are set but the yolk still feels bouncy, they are done.
9. To assemble the dish, put one half of each muffin on a plate, top with some spinach, then ham, then the poached eggs and pour the hollandaise over the top. (If the hollandaise has gone cold, simply reheat it by popping the bowl back over the pan and gently heating it through, whisking.) Sprinkle with the cayenne pepper and serve.

Carbs 54.7g

Calories 461

Fat 12.9g

Protein 26.7g

Raspberry Crumpet French Toast

This breakfast is a real indulgence, but it won't affect your fitness goals. High in protein, these crispy crumpets are topped with a sweet maple-raspberry compote and delicious salted caramel crème fraîche.

SERVES 2

60ml milk (of your choice)
1 scoop vanilla protein powder
1 tbsp granulated sweetener
2 large free-range eggs
1 tsp vanilla extract
4 crumpets
1 tbsp maple syrup
130g frozen raspberries
20g low-fat spread
2 tbsp half-fat salted caramel crème fraîche (use fat-free yoghurt, if you prefer)

1. In a rectangular oven dish (or shallow bowl), whisk together the milk, protein powder, sweetener, eggs and vanilla extract until combined.
2. Soak the crumpets in the egg mixture for 2–3 minutes on each side.
3. While the crumpets are soaking, place the maple syrup, frozen raspberries and a splash of water in a small saucepan and pop over a medium–low heat for around 5 minutes, or until thick and syrupy.
4. Melt the low-fat spread in a non-stick frying pan over a medium heat and fry the crumpets for no longer than 3 minutes per side.
5. Serve the crispy crumpets with the raspberry compote and dollops of the salted caramel crème fraîche.

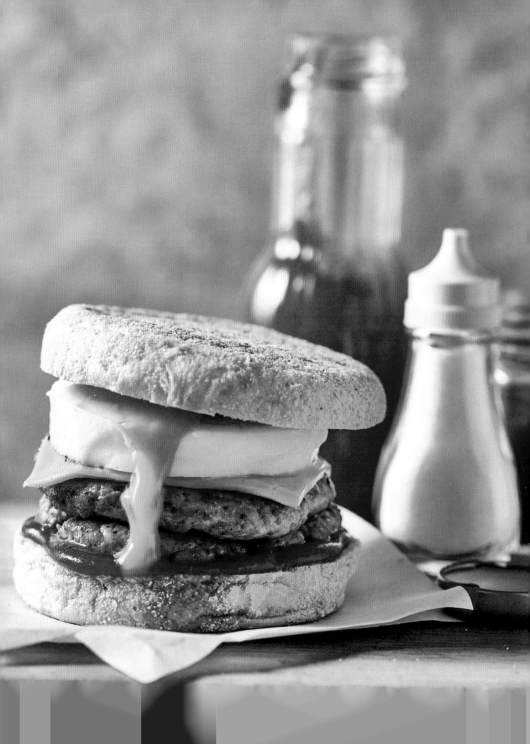

Carbs 31.5g	
Calories 329	
Fat 9.8g	
Protein 34.6g	

Double Sausage and Egg Muffins

You could be fooled into thinking this is the real thing – but it's not! High in protein and low in calories … your fitness plan will thank you for spending a short amount of time making your own.

SERVES 2

250g 5-per-cent-fat pork mince
½ tsp dried sage
½ tsp garlic granules
½ tsp onion powder
½ tsp sea salt
½ tsp freshly ground black pepper
Low-calorie cooking spray
2 reduced-fat cheese singles
2 free-range eggs
2 English muffins
Your favourite sauce, to serve

1. In a large bowl, use your hands to mix the pork mince with the dried sage, garlic granules, onion powder, sea salt and black pepper until well combined. Shape into four thin, round patties.
2. Spray a non-stick frying pan around ten times with the cooking spray and place over a medium–high heat.
3. Fry your patties for about 2 minutes on each side until golden and cooked through.
4. Pop the cheese singles on top of two of the patties and allow to melt. Leave in the pan to keep warm while you make the eggs.
5. Oil a cookie cutter and a non-stick frying pan with cooking spray.
6. Place the cookie cutter in the pan and heat over a medium–high heat. Crack the egg inside the cookie cutter and fry until the egg is cooked.
7. Halve the English muffins (and toast them if liked) and add two sausage patties (one with cheese and one without) to each muffin and then finish with the egg on top. Drizzle with your preferred sauce.

Carbs 6.7g

Calories 391

Fat 31.4g

Protein 21.6g

Chorizo and Egg Baked Avocado

This is a great low-carb, high-fat Mexican breakfast, which will have your taste buds tingling before it's even 10am!

SERVES 1
1 small avocado (ripe)
2 free-range eggs
50g chorizo, diced
Small handful of fresh
   coriander leaves
Sea salt
Freshly ground black
   pepper

1. Preheat the oven to 200°C/400°F/Gas 6.
2. Slice your avocado in half and remove the stone. Scoop out a good amount of the flesh to create a larger hole for the egg to sit in. (Make sure to use the leftover avocado for making guacamole or spreading over toast as a snack.)
3. Place the avocados on a baking tray and crack the eggs into the avocado holes. Bake for 15–20 minutes until the egg whites have set.
4. While the egg avocados are baking, fry the chorizo in a small, non-stick frying pan over a medium heat for 5 minutes until golden and cooked through. You shouldn't need any oil, as the natural oils from the chorizo will release when they are frying.
5. When the egg avocados have baked, spoon over the chorizo, season with sea salt and black pepper and tear over the coriander leaves.

Carbs 21.8g

Calories 359

Fat 9.7g

Protein 38.8g

Healthy Full English

This breakfast contains all the essential elements of a good fry-up, only it's much lower in calories. There's nothing 'bad' here, so you can enjoy this whenever you like. It would also make the perfect mid-week dinner.

SERVES 1

½ onion, finely chopped
Low-calorie cooking spray
1 garlic clove, finely
    chopped
1 tsp smoked paprika
½ tsp tomato purée
200g chopped tomatoes
    (½ 400g tin)
200g cannellini beans
    (½ 400g tin)
100g cherry tomatoes
    on the vine
100g chestnut mushrooms
2 chicken chipolatas
2 reduced-fat bacon
    medallions
1 free-range egg
Sea salt
Freshly ground black
    pepper

1. Preheat the oven to 190°C/375°F/Gas 5.
2. In a small saucepan, fry the onion with a few sprays of low-calorie cooking spray for 2–3 minutes over a medium heat until softened.
3. Add the garlic and fry for a further minute, then stir in the smoked paprika and tomato purée and fry for about 20 seconds.
4. Add the chopped tomatoes and cannellini beans and season with sea salt and black pepper. Simmer over a low heat while you get on with the rest.
5. Place the tomatoes, mushrooms and sausages on a baking tray and spray with a few sprays of cooking spray. Pop in the oven for 12–15 minutes until the tomatoes are blistered and the sausages are browned and cooked through.
6. Meanwhile, either fry or grill the bacon medallions according to the packet instructions.
7. Half fill another saucepan with water, bring to the boil and, once boiling, swirl it with the end of a wooden spoon to create a small whirlpool in the water. Crack the eggs, turn the heat off and leave for 3–4 minutes. To check if the eggs are cooked, lift one out of the water with a slotted spoon and if the whites are set but the yolk still feels bouncy, they are done.
8. Plate up and serve.

Carbs 40g

Calories 320

Fat 10g

Protein 16g

Egg Boats

This quick and easy recipe is so delicious it can be eaten for breakfast, lunch or dinner. Because let's face it, there's nothing like breakfast for dinner.

SERVES 1

1 sweet potato (about 200g uncooked)
2 cherry tomatoes
A few spinach leaves
2 free-range eggs
Sea salt
Freshly ground black pepper
A few snipped chives, to garnish (optional)

1. Prick holes in the sweet potato with a fork and microwave for 6–7 minutes until soft.
2. Once softened, slice in half and scoop out some of the insides to make enough room for the eggs. (Don't waste the scooped out potato, enjoy it as a snack as you cook).
3. Wrap the potato in foil (so the eggs don't spill out), then drop the spinach and tomatoes into the hollow, crack in the eggs and season well with sea salt and black pepper.
4. Place under the grill for 5–10 minutes until the egg is cooked just how you like it. Garnish with snipped chives if liked.

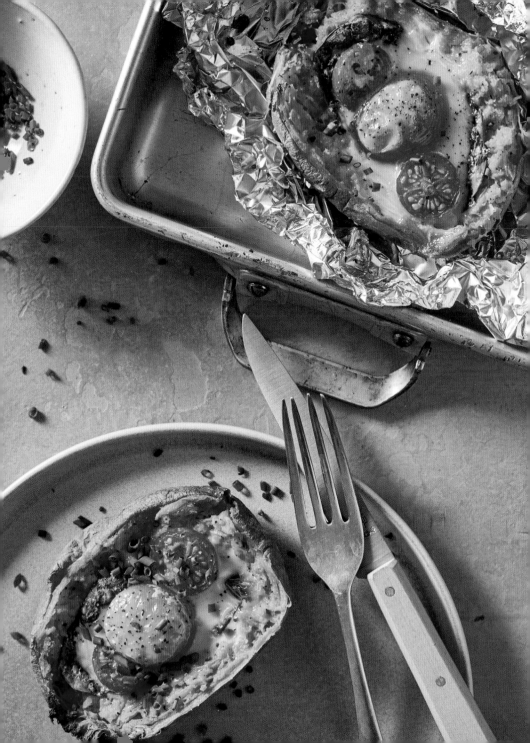

Carbs 26.7g

Calories 374

Fat 18g

Protein 24.4g

Shakshuka (Baked Eggs)

The word 'shakshuka' means 'a mixture' in Arabic, and we think that this dish is a mixture of miracles! It is spicy, sweet and warming and a perfect way to begin the weekend.

SERVES 2

1 tsp olive oil
1 onion, finely sliced
1 red pepper, deseeded and finely sliced
1 yellow pepper, deseeded and finely sliced
4 garlic cloves, finely sliced
1 tsp ground cumin
½ tsp ground cinnamon
1 tsp smoked paprika
1 tsp tomato purée
1 × 400g tin chickpeas, drained and rinsed
1 × 400g tin chopped tomatoes
1 tsp honey
1 tsp balsamic vinegar
Large handful of curly-leaf kale
4 free-range eggs
½ bunch fresh coriander leaves
60g feta
Sea salt
Freshly ground black pepper

1. In a large saucepan (preferably a high-sided, non-stick frying pan), heat the olive oil over a medium heat.
2. Add the onion and peppers and fry for 4–5 minutes until softened. Add the garlic and fry for a further 2 minutes.
3. Sprinkle over the spices and stir until the vegetables are well coated. Continue to fry, stirring constantly, for 1 minute.
4. Add the tomato purée, chickpeas, chopped tomatoes, honey, balsamic vinegar, kale and 100ml water, giving it a good stir to combine. Season with sea salt and black pepper to taste, then bring to a simmer and leave to cook gently for 5–7 minutes until the sauce has thickened.
5. Make four wells in the mixture with the back of a wooden spoon and crack an egg into each one.
6. Pop a lid on the pan and let the eggs steam for about 4–5 minutes until the whites have set, but the yolks are still runny.
7. Scatter with the fresh coriander, crumble the feta cheese over the top and serve.

TOP TIP: this works well with some toasted bread rubbed with a sliced garlic clove to dip in and mop up all of the delicious juices.

Carbs 42.3g	
Calories 346	
Fat 13.6g	
Protein 10.7g	

Sweet Potato Hash Browns

Sweet potatoes are full of nutrients, so we thought we would take the much-loved hash brown and make it way healthier. This high-protein breakfast will leave you feeling fuelled for hours.

SERVES 2

3 free-range eggs
200g sweet potato, coarsely grated
1 tsp garlic granules
1 tsp onion powder
1 tbsp olive oil
Small handful of fresh chives, finely sliced
Sea salt
Freshly ground black pepper

1. Crack one of the eggs into a large bowl and add the sweet potato, garlic granules, onion powder and a good pinch of sea salt and black pepper. Use your hands to mix together until well combined. Form into four flat discs of sweet potato mixture.
2. In a non-stick frying pan, heat the olive oil over a medium heat and fry the hash browns gently for about 3 minutes on each side until they are crispy and turning golden.
3. Half fill a saucepan with water, bring to the boil and, once boiling, swirl it with the end of a wooden spoon to create a small whirlpool. Crack the remaining eggs in, turn the heat off and leave to cook for 3–4 minutes, depending on how you like your eggs cooked.
4. Serve the hash browns with a poached egg and the chives sprinkled over the top. Add extra sea salt and black pepper on top of your eggs, if desired.

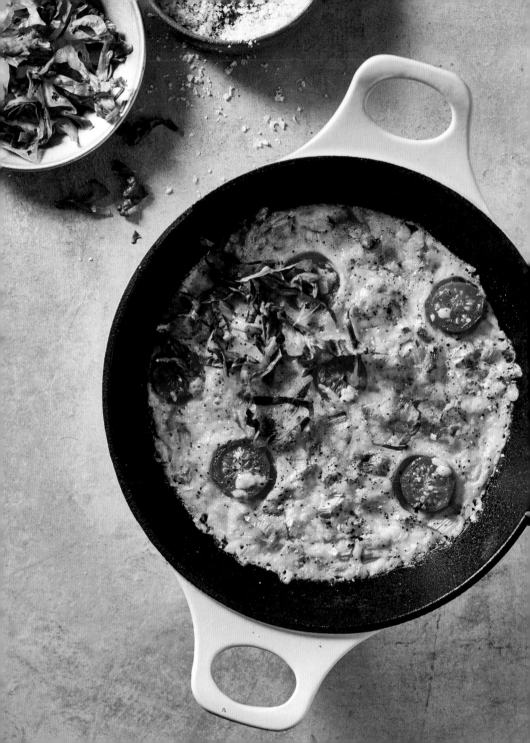

Carbs 20.7g

Calories 312

Fat 13.8g

Protein 38.5g

BLT Frittata

This delicious protein-packed frittata doesn't need to be reserved just for breakfast – this is a meal you can come back to at any time of the day. Add your favourite vegetables and protein or whatever is leftover in your fridge.

SERVES 1

Low-calorie cooking spray
2 smoked bacon medallions, sliced into strips
4 spring onions, sliced
5 cherry tomatoes, halved
2 large free-range eggs
1 large free-range egg white
50g low-fat cottage cheese
10g reduced-fat Cheddar, grated
1 large lettuce leaf (or rocket leaves for extra flavour), shredded
Sea salt
Freshly ground black pepper

1. Preheat the oven to 200°C/400°F/Gas 6.
2. Heat a non-stick ovenproof frying pan over a medium–high heat and add a few sprays of low-calorie cooking spray. Fry the bacon, spring onions and cherry tomatoes until the spring onions have softened and the bacon is beginning to turn golden.
3. Meanwhile, beat the eggs and egg white together until combined. Mix through the cottage cheese.
4. Keeping the heat of the pan high, pour in the eggs, ensuring the bottom of the pan is evenly coated. Leave this to fry for 2 minutes until the bottom of the egg has set. Sprinkle over the grated cheese, some black pepper and some sea salt.
5. Pop the pan in the oven for around 5 minutes, or until the egg has completely cooked through and set.
6. Sprinkle over the shredded lettuce to serve.

FAKEAWAYS

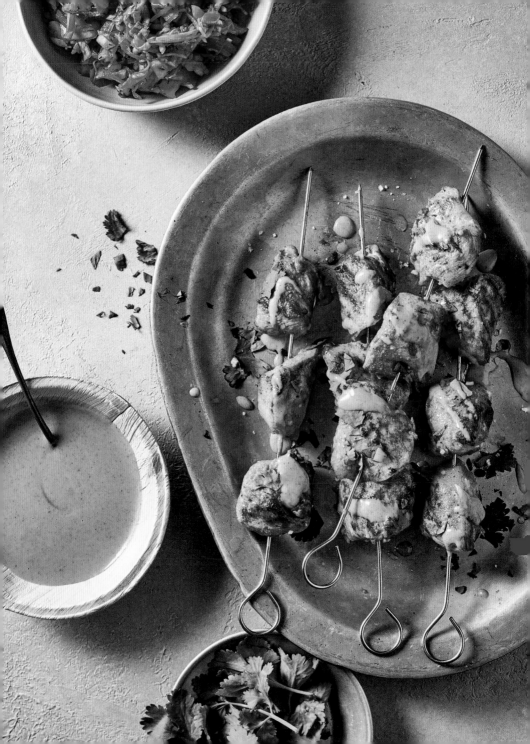

Carbs 14.4g

Calories 338

Fat 15.7g

Protein 39.2g

Quick Chicken Satay Skewers

I could have this homemade satay sauce on virtually anything – it's that good! But this recipe of skewered grilled chicken pairs perfectly with the creamy, sweet sauce. Serve alongside a delicious slaw or crunchy salad.

**SERVES 2
(MAKES 4 SKEWERS)**

FOR THE SKEWERS
2 garlic cloves, finely
   grated
1 tsp curry powder
2 tsp maple syrup
½ tsp turmeric
1 tsp low-sodium
   soy sauce
2 boneless, skinless
   chicken breasts, cut
   into bite-sized chunks
Freshly chopped
   coriander leaves,
   to garnish (optional)

**FOR THE SATAY
DIPPING SAUCE**
2 tbsp smooth peanut
   butter
1 tsp maple syrup
150ml tinned light
   coconut milk
1 tbsp low-sodium
   soy sauce
1 tbsp curry powder

1. Combine the garlic, curry powder, maple syrup, turmeric and soy sauce in a medium bowl.
2. Add the chicken to the bowl and stir to combine. Cover and place in the fridge for 10 minutes.
3. To make the satay sauce, warm all the ingredients in a saucepan over a low heat, whisking frequently to ensure a smooth sauce (do not allow it to boil). Set aside, ready for dipping.
4. Remove the chicken from the fridge and carefully push on to skewers.
5. Preheat the grill to high.
6. Place the skewers on a wire rack under a hot grill for 10–15 minutes until cooked through (when it's no longer pink and the juices run clear). You will need to turn them every now and again to ensure they are evenly cooked. Remove from the grill and garnish with coriander, if using, and serve with the dipping sauce.

TOP TIP: if using wooden skewers, place them in a bowl of water to soak (this will prevent them from burning in the oven).

Carbs 43.2g

Calories 592

Fat 25.8g

Protein 42.4g

Chock-a-block Nachos

This is my idea of a treat meal – but it's still below 600 calories! It is a deliciously layered nacho dish with a smoky BBQ ragu and melting mozzarella.

SERVES 4
(OR 6, AS A SIDE)
Low-calorie cooking spray
500g lean beef mince
1 large onion, finely sliced
1 red pepper, deseeded
  and finely sliced
3 garlic cloves, finely
  chopped
1 tbsp smoked paprika
½ tsp ground cumin
1 tbsp tomato purée
1 tbsp BBQ sauce
1 tbsp tomato ketchup
1 × 400g tin chopped
  tomatoes
1 chicken stock pot
200g salted tortilla chips
240g ball reduced-fat
  mozzarella, torn into
  strips
1 small red onion, finely
  chopped
Handful of fresh coriander
½ avocado, cut into slices
Sea salt
Freshly ground black
  pepper

1. Spray a good amount of cooking spray over a large, non-stick frying pan. Place over a medium–high heat and add the beef mince. Cook until it is browned all over, then keep stirring for about 10 minutes until it begins to crackle. Once the mince has caramelised and is a deep golden colour, use a slotted spoon to remove it from the pan and set aside.

2. Reduce the heat to medium, add the onion and red pepper and fry for 3–4 minutes until softened. Add the garlic and fry for a further minute. Add the smoked paprika and ground cumin and stir until the vegetables are coated.

3. Stir through the tomato purée, BBQ sauce and tomato ketchup and then pour over the chopped tomatoes, chicken stock pot and 100ml water. Return the mince to the pan and stir through. Bring to the boil, then reduce the heat to low. Leave to simmer gently for 40–45 minutes until most of the liquid has evaporated (you don't want the ragu to be watery, as this will make the tortilla chips soggy). Season with sea salt and black pepper.

4. Preheat the oven to 190°C/375°F/Gas 5.

5. Arrange half the tortilla chips on a large baking tray and top with half the ragu, half the mozzarella and half the chopped red onion.

6. Lay the rest of the tortilla chips on top and spoon over the remaining ragu, mozzarella and red onion. Sprinkle over the coriander leaves and top with the avocado.

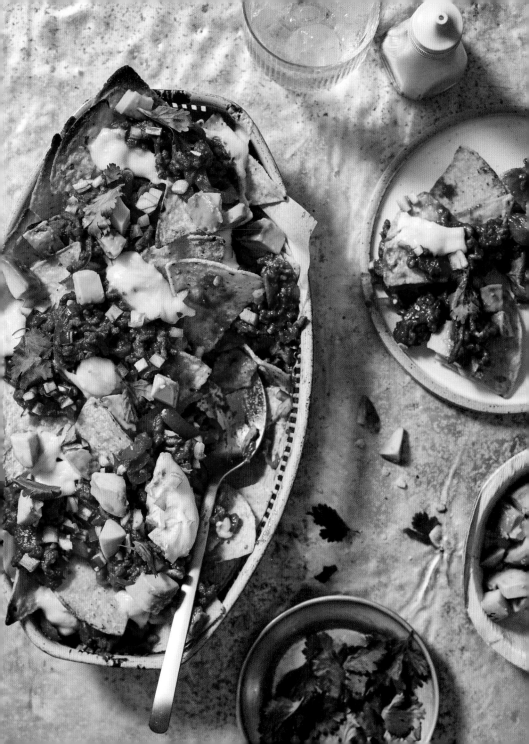

Carbs 46.9g

Calories 357

Fat 6.2g

Protein 27.3g

Fish-finger Sandwiches

The ultimate lunch or snack! Will you have yours with this amazing homemade tartare sauce, a dollop of tomato ketchup – or both? Decisions, decisions.

SERVES 2

200g cod loin, cut into
  finger-sized pieces
20g plain flour
1 free-range egg, beaten
50g cornflakes, crushed in
  a ziplock bag
4 slices white bread
Salad leaves, to serve
  (optional)

**FOR THE TARTARE
SAUCE**

1 tbsp light mayonnaise
1 tbsp fat-free yoghurt
1 tbsp capers, chopped
1 tbsp gherkins, chopped
  (optional)
Juice of 1 lemon
Sea salt
Freshly ground black
  pepper

1. Preheat the oven to 190°C/375°F/Gas 5 and line a baking tray with non-stick baking paper.
2. Grab three plates, placing the flour on the first, the beaten egg on the second and the crushed cornflakes on the third.
3. Gently pat the fish dry with kitchen paper. Dredge a piece of fish in the flour and pat off any excess.
4. Now add the fish to the egg, ensuring the entire finger is coated.
5. Lastly, add the fish to the cornflakes, rolling it to ensure it is fully coated in the crumbs.
6. Place the fish finger on the lined baking tray and continue the process until you have eight coated fish fingers ready to bake.
7. Pop these in the oven on a high rack and bake for 12–15 minutes until the fish is flaky and cooked and the cornflake crumb is golden.
8. While your fish fingers are baking, make the tartare sauce by simply mixing all the ingredients together.
9. Serve the fish fingers on white bread with a good dollop of tartare sauce and some salad, if you like.

Carbs 46.4g

Calories 352

Fat 14g

Protein 9.6g

Dough Balls with Garlic Butter

Keep your pizza – we're here for chewy, crispy and buttery dough balls! This recipe takes a little longer in preparation time, but trust us, it's worth it.

**MAKES 20 BALLS
(4 PER PERSON)**
325g strong white bread flour, plus extra for kneading and rolling
10g Parmesan, grated
1 × 7g sachet dried fast-action yeast
1½ tbsp olive oil
1 tsp sea salt
250ml warm water
Low-calorie cooking spray

FOR THE GARLIC BUTTER
3 garlic cloves
110g low-fat butter
½ tsp sea salt

1. Sift the flour into a large bowl along with the Parmesan. On one side of the bowl, add the yeast and olive oil and on the other side, add the salt.
2. Begin mixing with a wooden spoon or your hands until combined. Add the water gradually, mixing constantly, until it forms a dough.
3. Tip the dough ball on to a floured surface and knead for 5 minutes until smooth and stretchy. Return the dough ball to the large bowl and cover with a damp tea towel or cling film and leave in a warm place for 1 hour until doubled in size.
4. Punch the dough down until it has deflated, then tip on to a floured surface and knead lightly for 30 seconds. Divide the dough into 20 smaller balls. Between floured hands, gently roll the balls until they are even and neat.
5. Spray a large baking tray with low-calorie cooking spray and smear with your fingers to grease all over. Place the balls on the tray, roughly 2–3cm apart, giving them enough space to rise.
6. Cover the tray loosely with a tea towel or cling film and leave to sit for 20 minutes. Preheat the oven to 200°C/400°F/Gas 6.
7. To make the garlic butter, simply place the ingredients in a small blender and blitz until smooth.
8. After the 20 minutes, remove the tea towel or cling film and bake the dough balls for 20–25 minutes in the oven until golden and hollow.
9. As soon as the dough balls are cooked, spread some of the butter over to melt and serve the rest on the side for extra dipping!

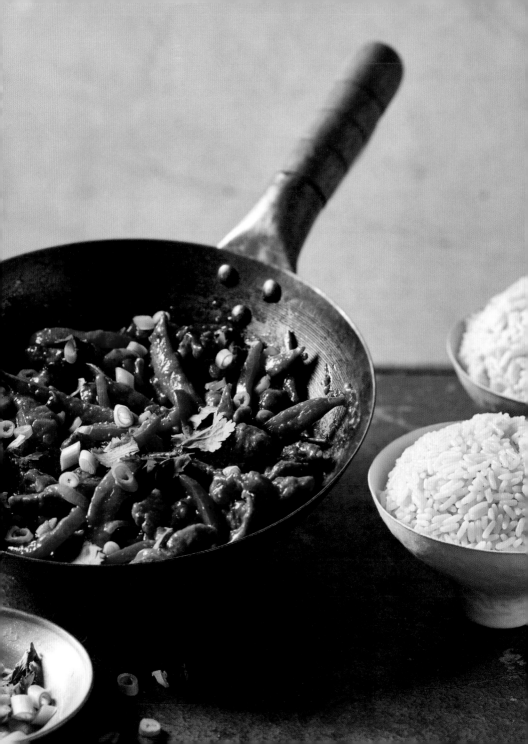

Carbs 26.2g

Calories 487

Fat 13.7g

Protein 61g

Beef in Black Bean Sauce

This dish is ready in no time and is full of protein, making it a great, healthy post-workout meal or even just a weekend fakeaway.

SERVES 2

1 tsp olive oil
1 tsp cornflour
350g beef stir-fry strips
1 onion, sliced
1 red pepper, deseeded
 and sliced
Low-calorie cooking spray
150g sugar snap peas
3 garlic cloves, finely
 grated
Thumb-sized piece of
 fresh ginger, finely
 grated
250g black bean cooking
 sauce
½ bunch fresh coriander
 leaves
2 spring onions, finely
 sliced
Sea salt
Freshly ground black
 pepper
Boiled rice, to serve

1. In a large, non-stick frying pan (or wok), heat the olive oil over a high heat. Season the cornflour with salt and pepper and rub all over the meat to lightly coat it.
2. Once the oil is very hot, add the beef and stir-fry for 3–4 minutes until browned all over. Remove from the pan and pop on a plate.
3. Add the onion and red pepper to the pan and stir-fry for 2–3 minutes until beginning to soften (you can add some low-calorie cooking spray to the pan if it seems a little dry). Add the sugar snaps and fry for a further minute.
4. Add the garlic and ginger and fry for a further minute. Pour in the black bean sauce, along with a splash of water and stir well.
5. Return the beef to the pan and leave the mixture to bubble away over a medium–low heat until the beef is cooked through.
6. Serve with the fresh coriander leaves and spring onions sprinkled over the top, along with some boiled rice.

Carbs 30.3g

Calories 371

Fat 15.5g

Protein 29.1g

Crispy Duck and Pancakes

Don't bother with the takeaway – this recipe is much healthier, and you will be so proud after you've made it!

SERVES 2
(3 PANCAKES PER PERSON)
2 duck legs
2 tbsp Chinese five-spice powder
2 tbsp hoisin sauce, plus extra to serve
2 tsp runny honey
6 Chinese pancakes
½ cucumber, finely sliced into matchsticks
4 spring onions, finely sliced into strands

TO SERVE
Hoisin sauce
Prawn crackers (optional)

1. Preheat the oven to 170°C/325°F/Gas 3.
2. Pat the duck legs dry with some kitchen paper and then poke the skin with a cocktail stick or skewer about ten times on each one. This will help the excess fat to cook out of the legs as they bake.
3. Rub the five-spice powder all over the legs, spoon over the hoisin sauce and drizzle with honey.
4. Bake for 1½ hours until charred, crispy, cooked through and easily shredded from the bone. Set the duck legs aside to rest for 10 minutes.
5. Take two forks and shred the skin and meat off the duck legs. Pile the shredded meat on to the pancakes with the cucumber, spring onions and extra hoisin sauce to serve.

Carbs 24.1g

Calories 153

Fat 1.6g

Protein 4.3g

Giant Baked Spring Rolls

There's no need for spring rolls to be a side dish – these are the main event. And because they are baked in the oven instead of deep-fried, they don't use any oil.

**SERVES 2
(4 LARGE ROLLS)**

200g mixed vegetables (e.g. cabbage, red pepper, carrots, spring onion, beansprouts), finely shredded

Thumb-sized piece of fresh ginger, finely grated

2 garlic cloves, finely grated

1 tsp Chinese five-spice powder

3 tsp low-sodium soy sauce

4 sheets filo pastry

80g straight-to-wok noodles

16 king prawns, cooked

1 egg, beaten

Low-calorie cooking spray

1 tsp sesame seeds

Sea salt

Freshly ground black pepper

1. Preheat the oven to 180°C/350°F/Gas 4.
2. Place the vegetables, ginger, garlic, five-spice powder and soy sauce in a large bowl and mix thoroughly. Season with salt and black pepper. Divide the mixure into 50g portions.
3. Lay out 1 sheet of filo pastry on a clean tea towel. Place 50g of the spiced vegetable mix in a strip at one end. Top with 20g of the noodles and four prawns.
4. Brush some beaten egg along the edges of the pastry sheet. Fold both edges over the filling, then roll up tightly into a large spring roll. Seal the long edge with some more beaten egg.
5. Continue with the remaining mixture and pastry until you have four large spring rolls.
6. Pop the spring rolls on a baking tray and spray a few times with cooking spray.
7. Sprinkle over the sesame seeds and bake for about 20–25 minutes until golden and crisp.

Cheat's Chicken Katsu Curry

FOR THE CHICKEN

2 tbsp plain flour

1 large free-range egg, beaten

60g cornflakes, crushed in a ziplock bag

2 boneless, skinless chicken breasts, bashed with a rolling pin to just over 1cm thick

½ bunch fresh coriander leaves, torn, to serve

1 red chilli, deseeded and finely sliced, to serve

FOR THE SAUCE

1 tsp olive oil

1 onion, finely diced

3 garlic cloves, finely grated

Thumb-sized piece of fresh ginger, peeled and grated

1 tbsp plain flour

1 tbsp curry powder (mild or hot)

1 heaped tsp ground turmeric

1 tbsp low-sodium soy sauce

1 tsp white wine vinegar

250ml chicken stock

2 small tsp honey or maple syrup

FOR THE RED ONION PICKLE

1 large red onion, finely sliced

2 tbsp white wine vinegar

1 tsp sea salt

2 tbsp caster sugar

Crunchy leaves, to serve

The nation's favourite Japanese restaurant dish made healthy. We've teamed this crispy chicken with a sweet-and-sour red onion pickle, but you can add basmati rice if you prefer.

1. Preheat the oven to 200°C/400°F/Gas 6. Line a baking tray with non-stick baking paper.

2. To make the red onion pickle, simply place all the ingredients in a small bowl and add a splash of very hot kettle water. Leave to pickle while you get on with the rest of the dish. When ready to serve, use a fork to pick out the onion, allowing the excess water to drip off.

3. To make the curry sauce, heat the oil in a large saucepan and fry the onion over a low heat for 10–12 minutes until softened but not browned. Add the garlic and ginger and cook for 2 minutes. Stir in the flour and cook for another minute.

4. Add the remaining sauce ingredients and turn the heat up to medium. Simmer for 15 minutes until thickened. Taste and season if necessary. Keep warm.

5. Grab three plates, placing the flour on the first, the beaten egg on the second and the crushed cornflakes on the third.

6. Dip each chicken breast in the flour, shaking off any excess, then in the egg, ensuring they are fully coated. Dredge the breasts in the cornflakes, patting down to ensure they are evenly coated all over.

7. Pop the chicken breasts on the lined baking tray and cook in the oven for 25–30 minutes, flipping halfway through, until the chicken is piping hot and cooked through (when it is no longer pink and the juices run clear).

8. At this point, you can either blitz the curry sauce in a blender until smooth, pass it through a sieve or simply eat it as it is.

9. Slice the chicken breasts into thick pieces and transfer to plates or bowls. Pour over the curry sauce and top with the red onion pickle, torn coriander leaves and sliced chilli. Serve with crunchy salad leaves on the side or rice, if you like.

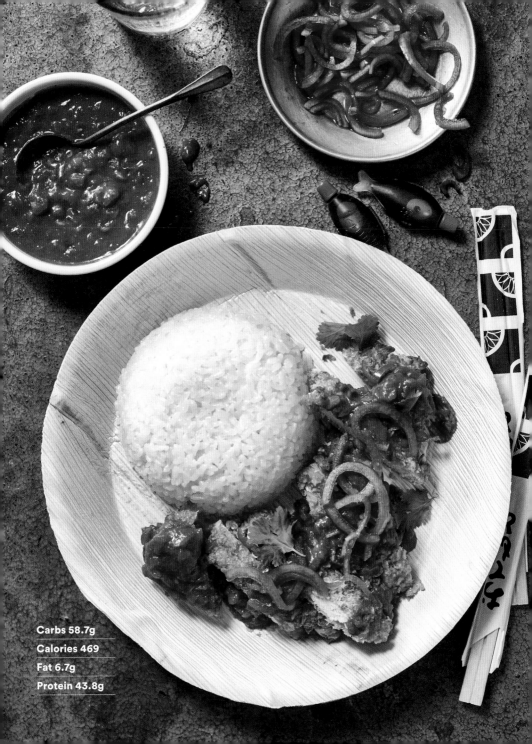

Carbs 58.7g

Calories 469

Fat 6.7g

Protein 43.8g

Carbs 28.6g	
Calories 495	
Fat 40.1g	
Protein 63.5g	

Five Girls Burger

The famous fast-food-joint burger is delicious, but if you want to make a much healthier version at home, here it is.

SERVES 2

400g extra-lean beef mince
1½ tsp garlic powder
1 tsp mustard powder
½ tbsp Worcestershire sauce
Low-calorie cooking spray
2 reduced-fat bacon medallions
2 reduced-fat cheese singles
2 sesame-seed burger buns, sliced
Sauce of your choice, to serve
1 Little Gem lettuce
Sea salt
Freshly ground black pepper

1. Place the beef mince, garlic powder, mustard and Worcestershire sauce in a mixing bowl, along with a good pinch of sea salt and black pepper and mix together with your hands.
2. Divide the mixture into four equal portions and form into balls. Place each ball between two pieces of non-stick baking paper and, using the palm of your hand, press down and squash into thin patties, roughly the size of your burger buns.
3. Preheat the grill to high.
4. Lightly oil a frying pan with low-calorie cooking spray and fry the bacon medallions until crispy. Remove and set aside.
5. Add the burger patties to the frying pan and cook over a high heat. Leave for 2–3 minutes before flipping.
6. In a second frying pan, gently toast the sliced buns until golden.
7. Once your burgers are cooked, place two of the patties on a baking tray (these will be your top patties) and lay a piece of bacon and a slice of cheese on each. Grill for a minute or so until the cheese is melting.
8. Add the sauce of your choice to the base of the buns, top with a plain patty and then the bacon and cheeseburgers, along with some lettuce leaves.

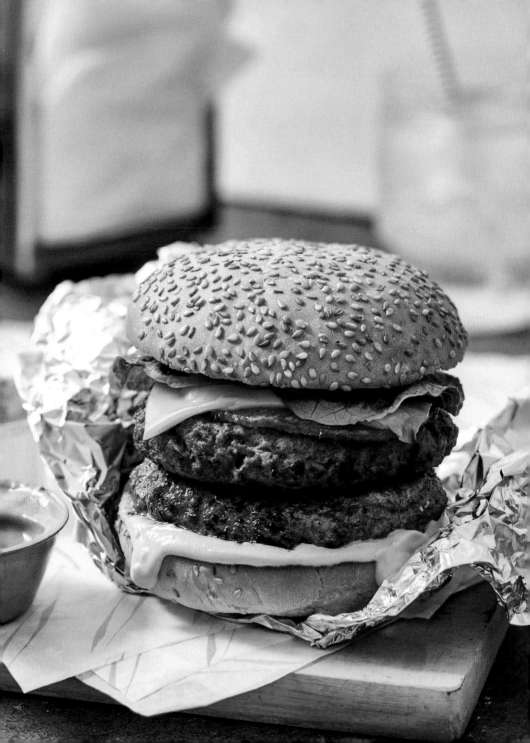

Carbs 23.2g

Calories 289

Fat 8.5g

Protein 30.6g

Lamb Rogan Josh

One of my favourite Indian takeaways – made lighter.

SERVES 2

2 tsp olive oil

1 red onion, sliced

1 red pepper, deseeded and sliced

300g extra-lean lamb, diced

3 garlic cloves, finely grated

Thumb-sized piece of fresh ginger, finely grated

1 × 35g sachet rogan josh spice mix

1 × 400g tin chopped tomatoes

1 x pouch microwave pilau rice

1. Heat the olive oil in a large, non-stick saucepan over a medium heat. Add the onion and red pepper and fry for about 5–7 minutes until golden and soft.
2. Add the lamb and continue frying until browned on all sides. Add the garlic and ginger, stirring, for a further minute.
3. Sprinkle over the spice mix and stir, ensuring everything is well coated. Fry for 1–2 minutes until fragrant.
4. Pour over the chopped tomatoes and a splash of water, then simmer over a low heat for 40–45 minutes.
5. Heat the rice according to the packet instructions and serve with the fragrant curry.

Carbs 47.5g	
Calories 551	
Fat 36.5g	
Protein 48.4g	

Bangin' Beef Enchiladas

These protein-packed enchiladas are easy to prepare, yet the result is so impressive. Pair with a simple salad for a wholesome dish.

SERVES 4

1 tbsp olive oil
500g extra-lean beef mince
1 large onion, finely diced
1 red pepper, deseeded and finely sliced
4 garlic cloves, finely chopped
1 tbsp smoked paprika
1 heaped tsp ground cumin
1 tsp ground cinnamon
½ tsp dried chilli flakes
3 tbsp chipotle chilli paste (available in most supermarkets)
100g tinned black beans, drained and rinsed
1 × 400g tin chopped tomatoes
1 tsp maple syrup
8 tortilla wraps
80g reduced-fat Cheddar, grated
100g reduced-fat mozzarella, grated
4 spring onions, finely sliced
Sea salt
Freshly ground black pepper

1. Preheat the oven to 200°C/400°F/Gas 6.
2. Pour the olive oil into a large, non-stick saucepan and bring to a medium heat. Add the mince and fry for about 5 minutes until browned all over.
3. Add the onion and red pepper and fry for 8–10 minutes until softened. Stir in the garlic and fry for a further 2 minutes.
4. Sprinkle in the spices and chilli flakes and stir well, cooking for a further minute.
5. Stir in the chipotle chilli paste, black beans, chopped tomatoes and maple syrup and season with salt and pepper. Bring to the boil and then reduce the heat and simmer for 25–30 minutes until thickened.
6. Fill each of the tortilla wraps with the smoky beef filling, reserving a quarter of it for the top.
7. Roll up the wraps and fold each end. Flip them over (so that the folded seams are on the bottom) and place in a roasting dish next to each other, snuggly.
8. Top with the remaining filling and then with the cheeses and bake for 20 minutes until golden and bubbling. Sprinkle over the spring onions and serve.

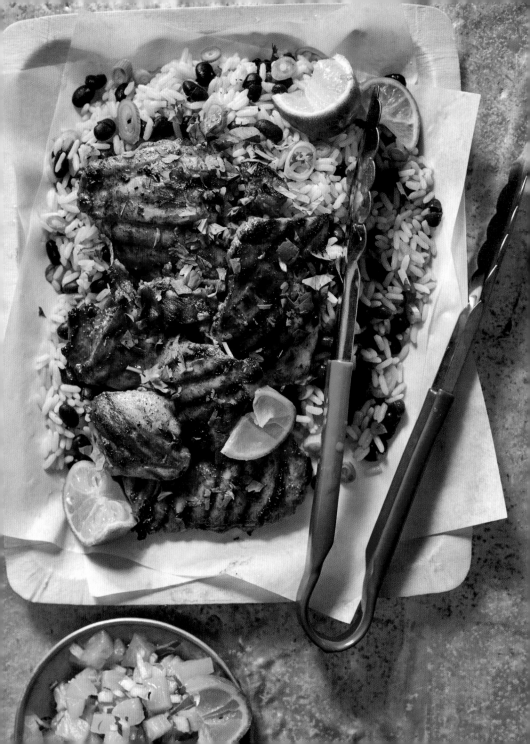

Carbs 66g

Calories 495

Fat 14g

Protein 23.1g

Jerk Chicken with Pineapple Salsa

Embrace the flavours of the Caribbean with this stunning jerk chicken recipe. Make sure to use some of the juice from the pineapple to give your salsa a sweet kick.

SERVES 4

1 tbsp light soy sauce
½ tbsp Worcestershire sauce
½ tbsp sugar-fee maple syrup
2 tsp sriracha
2 tbsp dried jerk spice mix
Juice of 1½ limes, plus wedges, to serve
3 garlic cloves, grated
Thumb-sized piece of fresh ginger, finely grated
4 chicken thighs
1 tbsp olive oil
2 pouches boil-in-the bag long-grain rice
1 × 400g tin black beans, drained and rinsed
4 spring onions, finely sliced
100g tinned pineapple, finely diced, juice reserved
2 red onions, finely diced
2 tbsp freshly chopped coriander leaves
Sea salt
Freshly ground black pepper

1. Preheat the oven to 200°C/400°F/Gas 6.
2. In a large mixing bowl, combine the soy sauce, Worcestershire sauce, maple syrup, sriracha, jerk spice mix, juice of 1 lime, garlic and ginger. Season with salt and pepper, then add the chicken thighs, coating them evenly in the marinade. Leave to marinate for at least 30 minutes (or overnight in the fridge for maximum flavour).
3. Lightly oil and heat a griddle or frying pan over a high heat. Remove the chicken from its marinating juices and cook for 2–3 minutes on either side until the skin is crisp and golden.
4. Transfer the chicken to a baking tray lined with non-stick baking paper and cook in the oven for 40 minutes, or until it is done (when no pink remains and the juices run clear).
5. Bring a pan of water to the boil and cook the rice according to the packet instructions. Drain, fluff with a fork and transfer to a serving dish. Mix through the black beans and spring onions.
6. To make the pineapple salsa, mix together the pineapple, red onions, remaining lime juice and a small splash of pineapple juice.
7. Serve the jerk chicken on a bed of rice and beans, along with a drizzle of pineapple salsa on each thigh and chopped coriander and wedges of lime in a large dish that everyone can dig into.

Carbs 35g

Calories 218

Fat 8g

Protein 4g

Sushi

We all love sushi, but it can be very expensive in a restaurant, so we've developed a cheaper (and healthier) version for you to enjoy from the comfort of your own home. You'll need some sushi rice, nori seaweed and a sushi mat (all available at large supermarkets and online) and your favourite fillings.

SERVES 2

50g sushi rice
1 small red onion, peeled and finely sliced
15ml white wine vinegar, plus 2 tbsp for the rice
60g cooked king prawns
1 tbsp teriyaki sauce
2 nori seaweed sheets
2 smoked salmon slices
1 avocado, thinly sliced
2 tsp sushi pickled ginger
¼ cucumber, sliced into thin matchsticks
2 spring onions, sliced into thin matchsticks
1 tsp wasabi paste
2 tbsp light mayonnaise
Light soy sauce, for dipping
½ tsp dried chilli flakes

1. Cook the rice according to the packet instructions. Once cooked, set aside to cool.
2. Place the sliced red onion in a bowl with the white wine vinegar and a dash of boiling water. Set aside while you make the rest.
3. In a small bowl, mix together the prawns and teriyaki sauce. Set aside to marinate.
4. Once the rice has cooled, gently stir in 2 tablespoons of white wine vinegar.
5. To assemble the sushi, lay one sheet of nori on a sushi mat with the lines of the mat horizontal in front of you.
6. With slightly wet hands, take a scoop of rice and spread it out over the nori (roughly the thickness of a pound coin), leaving a 2cm horizontal strip of nori uncovered at the top.
7. Lay the salmon in thin strips over the rice at the bottom of the nori square. Top with a strip of avocado slices and half the pickled ginger.
8. Starting at the bottom, use the sushi mat to roll the nori over the fillings, gradually moving the mat around the sushi roll and away from you. Once the sushi is rolled up almost to the strip of rice-free nori, dampen the seaweed with a little water to create a sticky seal and continue to use the mat to finish rolling up. Make sure to keep the sushi tightly rolled as you go to ensure it is firmly packed. When you've finished rolling, set the sushi tube on a plate, seal-side down.

9. Repeat, but this time using the cucumber and teriyaki prawns with some red onion, spring onions and the remaining pickled ginger.
10. Once both rolls are ready, use a sharp knife to cut into bite-sized pieces.
11. Mix together the wasabi paste and mayonnaise.
12. Serve the sushi with dipping bowls of wasabi mayonnaise and soy sauce mixed with the chilli flakes.

Salmon Biriyani

Carbs 32.1g

Calories 469

Fat 22.6g

Protein 32.4g

A traditional biryani takes a long time to cook, but not this one. I've made this really simple to cook midweek or at the weekend. Salmon is full of heart-healthy omega-3 fatty acids, which is great for supporting your skin and brain.

SERVES 4

300g basmati rice
1 tbsp olive oil
2 large onions, finely chopped
2 garlic cloves, finely chopped
1 tbsp grated fresh ginger
3 tbsp mild curry paste
600ml vegetable stock
150g frozen peas
200g baby spinach
4 cooked boneless, skinless salmon fillets
1 tbsp flaked almonds
½ bunch fresh coriander
Sea salt
Freshly ground black pepper

1. Rinse the rice in a sieve under cold water for a couple of minutes. Drain and set aside.
2. Heat the oil in a large frying pan (you'll need one with a lid) over a medium heat and gently fry the onions for 8–10 minutes until softened and slightly golden. Stir in the garlic and ginger and fry for a further 2 minutes.
3. Stir in the curry paste until loosened, then add the rice and stock. Bring the pan to the boil and reduce to a simmer. Pop the lid on and cook for 10 minutes.
4. Remove the lid, stir in the peas, then replace the lid and cook for a further 5 minutes.
5. Remove the pan from the heat, stir in the spinach and salmon and leave to sit for 5 minutes with the lid on.
6. Meanwhile, fry the flaked almonds in a dry pan over a medium heat until the toasted aromas are released.
7. Serve the biryani with the flaked almonds, some salt and pepper and fresh coriander sprinkled over the top.

Carbs 42.4g

Calories 424

Fat 10.6g

Protein 37.6g

Chicken Fajitas

Fajitas are the ultimate family dish – everyone can tuck in. I've made this one low calorie, using chicken-breast strips and packing in extra fresh vegetables. Special enough for a weekend feast, but quick enough for a midweek supper.

SERVES 4

400g chicken breast
   mini fillets
3 red onions, cut into
   wedges
2 red peppers, deseeded
   and cut into wedges
8 cherry tomatoes
1 red chilli, deseeded and
   finely sliced
1 tbsp ground cumin
1 tbsp smoked paprika
1 tbsp olive oil
Juice of 1 lime
8 mini tortilla wraps
60g salad leaves,
   e.g. rocket
Sea salt
Freshly ground black
   pepper

TO SERVE

Fresh coriander leaves
Fat-free crème fraîche
Tomato salsa or
   guacamole

1. In a large bowl, stir together the chicken, red onions, red peppers, cherry tomatoes, red chilli, ground cumin, paprika, olive oil and lime juice. Make sure everything is well coated. Season well with lots of sea salt and black pepper.

2. Heat a large, non-stick frying pan or a griddle pan over a very high heat. Once hot, add the chicken and vegetables and fry for 10 minutes until the chicken is cooked through (when it is no longer pink and the juices run clear) and the vegetables have begun to char slightly. Be careful not to move the ingredients around too much in the pan, as you want it to develop nice caramelised marks (for extra flavour!).

3. Load the tortilla wraps with the delicious smoky chicken and vegetables, crisp salad leaves and add your preferred toppings.

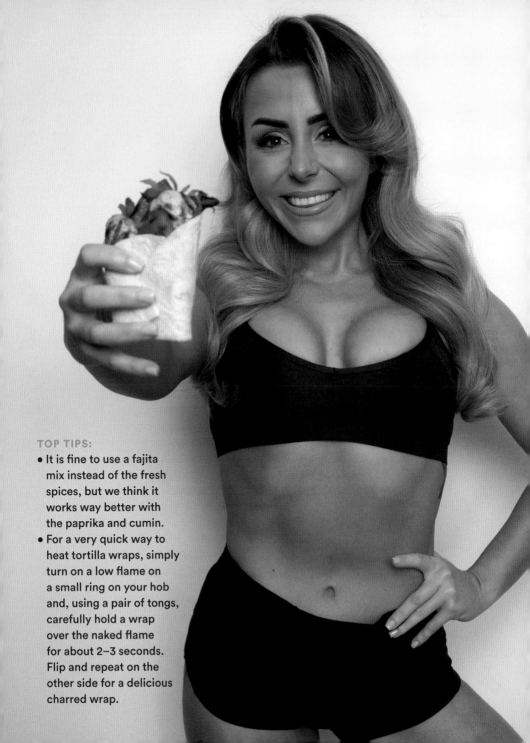

TOP TIPS:

- It is fine to use a fajita mix instead of the fresh spices, but we think it works way better with the paprika and cumin.
- For a very quick way to heat tortilla wraps, simply turn on a low flame on a small ring on your hob and, using a pair of tongs, carefully hold a wrap over the naked flame for about 2–3 seconds. Flip and repeat on the other side for a delicious charred wrap.

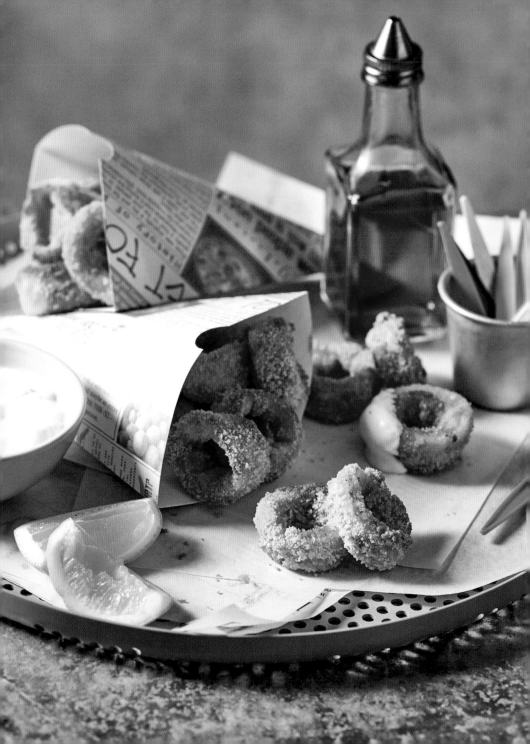

Easy Breaded Calamari

We all love crispy calamari and here is a healthy one for you to enjoy as a starter for four or a more substantial treat for two.

**SERVES 4
(AS A STARTER)**

80g plain flour
2 free-range eggs, beaten
150g breadcrumbs
¼ tsp sea salt, plus extra
   for sprinkling
¼ tsp freshly ground black
   pepper
300g squid rings (if
   using frozen, defrost
   according to packet
   instructions)
Pinch of cayenne
   pepper or paprika, for
   sprinkling (optional)
Lemon wedges, to serve

FOR THE DIPPING SAUCE

2 tbsp reduced-fat
   mayonnaise
1 tbsp fat-free yoghurt
1 garlic clove, finely
   grated
Juice of ½ lemon

1. Preheat the oven to 200°C/400°F/Gas 6. Line a baking tray with non-stick baking paper.
2. To make the dipping sauce, place all the ingredients in a bowl and mix together. Refrigerate until ready to use.
3. Place the plain flour, eggs and breadcrumbs in three separate bowls. Add the salt and pepper to the breadcrumbs.
4. Dip each squid ring into the flour, then the egg and finally the breadcrumbs, patting off any excess in between dipping in each bowl.
5. Lay each squid ring on the lined baking tray. Bake for 15 minutes until golden, piping hot and cooked through. Sprinkle with extra sea salt and the cayenne pepper or paprika (if using).
6. Serve with the dipping sauce and lemon wedges.

Carbs 45.5g

Calories 321

Fat 2.4g

Protein 30.2g

Sweet-and-Sour Chicken

This much-loved takeaway is usually full of fat and sugar, but by using the juice from the pineapple, I've made this fakeaway version much healthier. Will it become your Friday-night favourite?

SERVES 4

1 tbsp honey
Thumb-sized piece of
    fresh ginger, grated
3 garlic cloves, grated
1 tbsp low-sodium
    soy sauce
2 tbsp rice wine vinegar
2 tbsp reduced-salt
    tomato ketchup
1 × 425g tin pineapple,
    drained and juice
    reserved
2 tsp cornflour
Low-calorie cooking spray
    (aromatic version)
3 skinless, boneless
    chicken breasts, cut into
    large chunks
1 red pepper, deseeded
    and cut into chunks
    (similar in size to the
    chicken)
1 green pepper, deseeded
    and cut into chunks
    (similar in size to the
    chicken)
1 red onion, sliced
2 pouches microwave
    long-grain rice
1 tsp dried chilli flakes

1. In a small saucepan, mix together the honey, ginger, garlic, soy sauce, vinegar, ketchup and pineapple juice. Place over a low heat and gently cook for about 5–10 minutes.
2. Mix the cornflour with a splash of water in a small cup, stirring with a fork until it has dissolved into a paste. Add to the juice mixture and bring to the boil. As soon as it begins to boil, turn the heat to low and simmer for 2 minutes, stirring frequently.
3. Heat about ten sprays of the low-calorie cooking spray in a large, non-stick frying pan (or wok) and stir-fry the chicken chunks over a high heat until they are cooked through (when they are no longer pink and the juices run clear). Remove and set aside.
4. Add the peppers and red onion to the pan and stir-fry for 3 minutes until softened.
5. Return the chicken to the pan and reduce the heat. Pour in the sweet-and-sour sauce and heat through over a medium–low heat for a couple of minutes.
6. Heat the rice according to the packet instructions.
7. Serve the rice with the sweet-and-sour chicken spooned over the top, sprinkled with chilli flakes.

Carbs 19.8g

Calories 448

Fat 23.4g

Protein 38.7g

Quick Thai Green Chicken Curry

Instantly recognisable, this Thai green curry is spicy, creamy and full of the good stuff! It is much easier to make than you might think and is a definite crowd pleaser. I particularly love the aromatic taste – and if you can get your hands on sesame oil, definitely use it. I like this dish with new potatoes, but you could easily boil up some rice on the side instead.

SERVES 2

100g new potatoes, halved (or quartered if on the large side)

1 tsp toasted sesame oil (or just use olive oil)

1 onion, finely sliced

2 garlic cloves, finely chopped

1 red chilli, deseeded and finely chopped

3 tbsp Thai green curry paste

1 × 400ml tin light coconut milk

2 boneless, skinless chicken breasts, cut into large chunks

100g beansprouts

1 large handful of baby spinach

Juice of ½ lime, plus wedges, to serve (optional)

1 tsp fish sauce

½ bunch fresh coriander leaves

1. Boil the potatoes for about 5 minutes until cooked through. Drain and set aside.
2. Heat the oil in a medium, non-stick frying pan over a medium heat and fry the onion, garlic and chilli for about 3–5 minutes until softened and turning golden.
3. Add the curry paste and cook for a minute or so, stirring frequently.
4. Add the coconut milk and cook over a high heat until bubbling, then reduce the heat to medium–low and add the chicken, cooking for 5–6 minutes, or until completely cooked through (when it's no longer pink and the juices run clear).
5. Add the beansprouts, spinach, lime juice and fish sauce. Stir well and cook for a further 2 minutes until the spinach has wilted.
6. Add the new potatoes and serve with lots of fresh coriander and extra lime wedges, if desired.

Carbs 39.2g

Calories 448

Fat 20g

Protein 25.8g

Steak Bake Fakeaway

This is a convincing version of the nation's favourite pasty – high in protein and low in calories, it's a sensational substitute for the real thing!

SERVES 1

60g lean diced beef, cut into 1cm cubes

Low-calorie cooking spray

200ml boiling water

2 tbsp beef casserole seasoning mix

1 tsp balsamic vinegar

80g light puff pastry

1 small free-range egg, beaten

Freshly ground black pepper

1. Preheat the oven to 190°C/375°F/Gas 5.
2. Brown the beef in a non-stick pan over a high heat with about five sprays of cooking spray. Once browned all over, pour in the boiling water and the seasoning mix, stirring well until combined.
3. Stir through the balsamic vinegar and a decent amount of black pepper and turn the heat down. Leave to simmer for 2–3 minutes over a low heat until thickened.
4. Meanwhile, roll out the pastry on a lightly floured surface into two rectangles measuring roughly 10 x 20cm each. One rectangle will be for the top of the pasty and the other will be for the bottom.
5. Take one rectangle and brush egg around the edges. Spoon in the beef mixture (you probably won't need all of the juice), being careful not to let it spill over the sides too much.
6. Score two lines on the other rectangle with a sharp knife and place it on top, using a fork to press down the edges (this will stop the beef mixture from seeping out while it is baking). Brush some more beaten egg over the top.
7. Bake in the oven for 20 minutes until the pastry is golden and puffed up.

Carbs 28.2g

Calories 323

Fat 6.6g

Protein 30.4g

Speedy Chicken Tikka Masala

A chicken tikka masala is something we always come back to – perfect for midweek, this recipe is so simple and comes in at a fraction of the calories of the nation's favourite takeaway dish.

SERVES 4

1 tbsp olive oil
1 onion, finely sliced
1 red pepper, deseeded and finely sliced
3 boneless, skinless chicken breasts, cut into large chunks
3 garlic cloves, finely chopped
1 tsp finely grated fresh ginger
1½ tsp garam masala
1½ tsp medium chilli powder
1 tsp turmeric
2 tbsp tomato purée
1 × 400g tin chopped tomatoes
1 teaspoon maple syrup
4 tbsp low-fat yoghurt
2 pouches microwave basmati rice
Juice of ½ lemon
½ bunch fresh coriander leaves
Sea salt
Freshly ground black pepper

1. In a large frying pan, heat the olive oil over a medium heat and add the onion and red pepper. Fry for about 5 minutes until softened.
2. Add the chicken to the pan and fry over a medium–high heat for another 5 minutes until almost cooked through.
3. Add the garlic and ginger and stir, frying for a further minute. Add the garam masala, chilli powder and turmeric and cook for another minute until fragrant.
4. Stir in the tomato purée, chopped tomatoes and maple syrup, then fill the tomato tin a quarter full with water and add this to the pan. Bring to a simmer and cook for 8–10 minutes until the chicken is cooked through (when it's no longer pink and the juices run clear) and the sauce has slightly reduced. Stir through the yoghurt and season.
5. Heat the rice in the microwave according to the packet instructions.
6. When the curry is cooked, squeeze over the lemon juice, scatter over the fresh coriander leaves and serve.

Carbs 53.7g

Calories 511

Fat 11g

Protein 47.6g

Fried Chicken Burger

If you're looking for a healthy version of the nation's most famous takeaway fried chicken burger, look no further. This low-fat, crispy chicken alternative is guaranteed to put a big smile on your face. Just ask the Colonel.

SERVES 2

1 tbsp plain flour
1 free-range egg, beaten
½ tbsp sriracha
5 tbsp wholemeal breadcrumbs (or 20g cornflakes, lightly crushed)
½ tsp smoked paprika
½ tsp garlic powder
½ tsp chilli powder
½ tsp dried mixed herbs
½ tsp onion powder
½ tsp cayenne pepper
½ tsp ground ginger
2 boneless, skinless chicken breasts
Low-calorie cooking spray
2 burger buns
1 large tomato, sliced
1 Little Gem lettuce
Sea salt
Freshly ground black pepper

FOR THE SPICY MAYO

1 tbsp light mayonnaise
1 tbsp tomato ketchup
1 tsp malt vinegar
2 tsp sriracha

1. Preheat the oven to 200°C/400°F/Gas 6. Line a baking tray with non-stick baking paper.
2. Grab three bowls. Put the plain flour in the first one. Mix the beaten egg and sriracha together in the second one. Mix the breadcrumbs (or cornflakes), smoked paprika, garlic powder, chilli powder, dried herbs, onion powder, cayenne pepper and ground ginger with a pinch of salt and pepper in the third bowl.
3. Pat the chicken breasts dry, lay them on a work surface and dredge them in the plain flour until well coated all over, shaking off any excess.
4. Dip the breasts into the egg mixture and gently shake off any excess.
5. Finally, coat the chicken breasts in the spiced breadcrumbs (or cornflakes), ensuring they are completely coated. Spray all over with cooking spray.
6. Place the breasts on the lined baking tray and cook for 35–40 mixtures, flipping for the last 10 minutes of cooking.
7. While the chicken is cooking, prepare the spicy mayo by combining all the ingredients in a bowl.
8. In a dry frying pan, toast the bun halves over a low–medium heat until lightly golden.
9. Once the chicken is cooked through (when it is no longer pink and the juices run clear), assemble the burgers. Spread the base of the buns with a little of the spicy mayo, add tomato slices, some lettuce leaves and the crispy chicken on top.

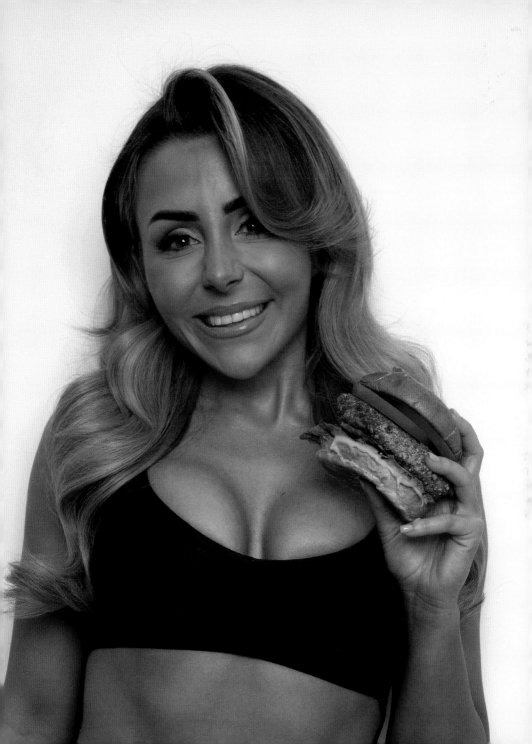

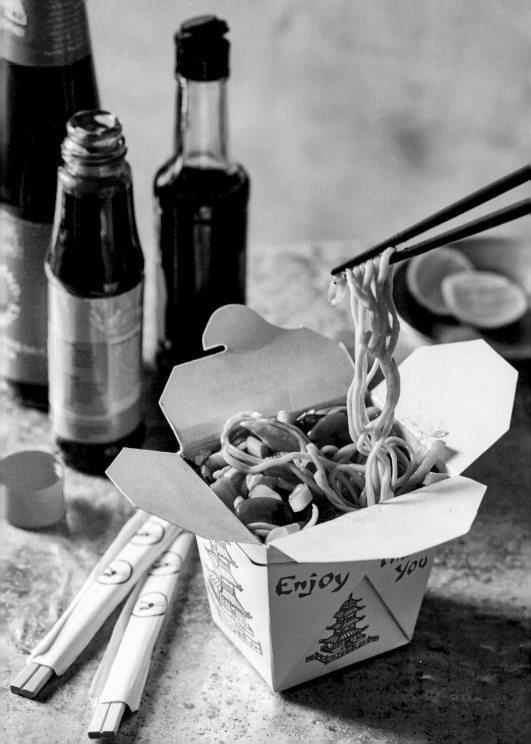

Carbs 56.7g

Calories 519

Fat 10.9g

Protein 48.4g

Spicy Drunken Noodles

This popular Thai dish will knock your socks off! Both sweet and sour, it is high in protein and low in fat.

SERVES 2

1 tbsp tomato ketchup

1 tbsp oyster sauce

2 tbsp low-sodium soy sauce

1 tsp fish sauce

Juice of 1 lime

100g dried egg noodles

1 tbsp garlic-infused olive oil

1 red onion, sliced

1 red pepper, deseeded and sliced

1 carrot, peeled and cut into wide matchsticks

1 red chilli, deseeded, if desired, and finely sliced

250g chicken breast mini fillets

50g beansprouts

200g pak choi, root removed and leaves sliced

3 spring onions, finely sliced

½ bunch fresh coriander leaves, torn

1. To make the sauce, place the ketchup, oyster sauce, soy sauce, fish sauce, lime juice and 1 tablespoon water in a small bowl and stir to combine. Set aside.
2. Cook the noodles in a pan of boiling water according to the packet instructions, then drain and set aside.
3. Pour the oil into a large, non-stick frying pan (or wok) over a high heat and add the onion, red pepper, carrot and red chilli. Stir-fry for 3 minutes until softened.
4. Add the chicken and stir-fry for a further 2–3 minutes until the chicken is almost cooked. Add the beansprouts, pak choi and noodles to the pan and stir-fry for 2 minutes.
5. Pour over the sauce and turn the heat down slightly. This will stop the ingredients frying and allow the sauce to coat everything. Stir well.
6. Serve with the spring onions and fresh coriander leaves sprinkled over the top.

Carbs 49.4g

Calories 422

Fat 13.5g

Protein 27.3g

Mexican Prawn Tacos with Quick Mango Salsa

A quick Mexican feast – made lighter with delicious crunchy prawns and a vibrant mango salsa.

SERVES 2

1 tbsp taco seasoning
1 tsp olive oil
240g fresh raw king prawns (or frozen)
1 small red onion, finely diced
100g fresh mango, finely diced
1 tbsp red wine vinegar
1 tsp maple syrup
½ bunch of fresh coriander
4 mini tortilla wraps
½ avocado, sliced
Lime wedges, to serve
Sea salt
Freshly ground black pepper

1. In a small bowl, mix together the taco seasoning, olive oil and a good amount of sea salt and black pepper. Add the prawns and mix until they are well coated. Set aside for a couple of minutes while you make the salsa.
2. In a small bowl, mix together the red onion, mango, red wine vinegar and maple syrup. Finely chop half the coriander and add to the bowl, along with some sea salt and black pepper. Mix well and set aside.
3. Heat a non-stick frying pan over a medium–high heat and, once hot, fry the prawns for 1–2 minutes on each side, or until pink all the way through.
4. Build the tacos by adding the prawns, then the avocado and finish by spooning over the delicious mango salsa. Serve with lime wedges and the remaining coriander.

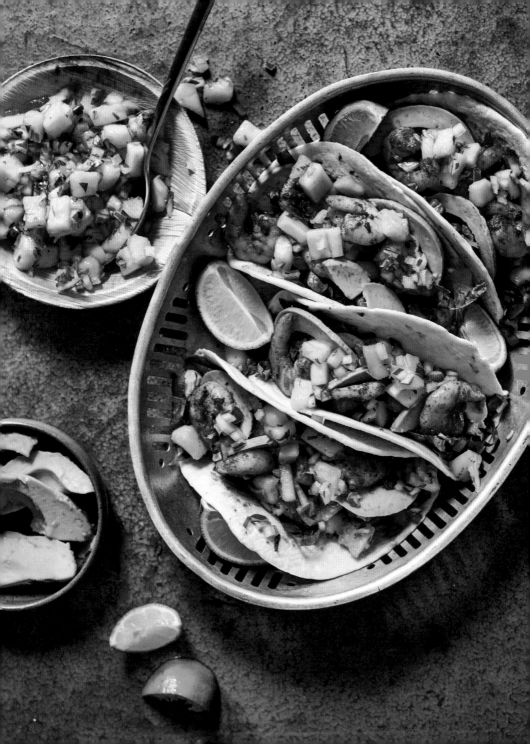

FAMILY CLASSICS

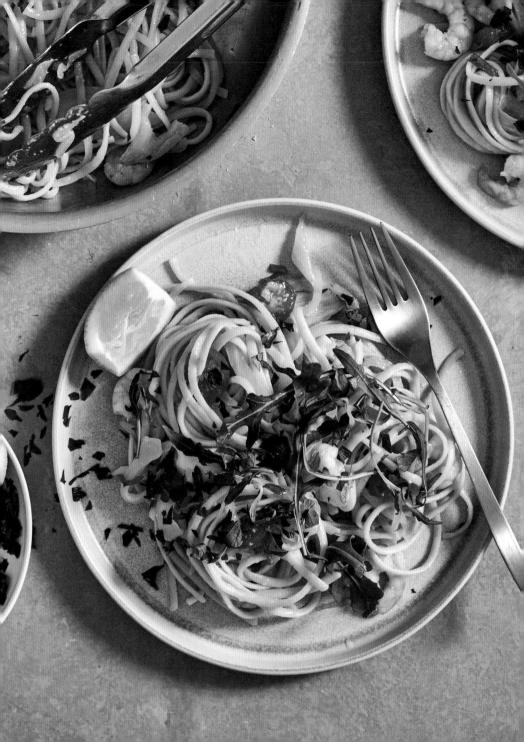

Chilli Prawn and Fennel Linguine

Prawns are a great source of protein, vitamin B and niacin, helping the body to produce energy. They are also low in fat, which makes for the perfect pasta dish. If you don't like fennel or fennel seeds, simply leave them out and add some extra onion instead.

SERVES 4
300g linguine
1 tsp olive oil
1 large fennel bulb, thinly sliced (or 1 heaped tbsp fennel seeds)
4 garlic cloves, thinly sliced or crushed
1 red chilli, deseeded and finely sliced or ½ tsp dried chilli flakes
1 onion, thinly sliced
10 cherry tomatoes, halved
330g raw king prawns
Juice of ½ lemon, plus lemon wedges to serve
Handful of fresh parsley
Handful of fresh rocket
Sea salt
Freshly ground black pepper

1. Fill a large pan with boiling water and add a good amount of salt. Bring to the boil over a medium heat. Boil the pasta according to the packet instructions.
2. Meanwhile, in a large, high-sided frying pan, heat the olive oil over a low–medium heat and fry the fennel (or fennel seeds), garlic, red chilli (or chilli flakes) and onion until softened, but not browned.
3. Add the tomatoes and prawns to the pan and turn the heat up slightly. You can add a splash of the pasta water and shake the pan to mix everything together.
4. When the pasta is cooked, drain and add to the prawns, along with the lemon juice and give everything a good toss. Taste and season with salt and pepper, if needed. Plate and top with the parsley, rocket and lemon wedges.

Carbs 56.7g

Calories 456

Fat 17g

Protein 32.7g

Spaghetti Bolognaise

Bolognese is arguably the ultimate pasta dish and we've made a really simple one here, so you can enjoy those authentic Italian flavours at home.

SERVES 4

1 tbsp olive oil
1 large onion, finely chopped
2 carrots, finely chopped
2 celery sticks, finely chopped
250g extra-lean beef mince
150g extra-lean pork mince
2 garlic cloves, finely chopped
100ml red wine
300ml tomato passata
1 tbsp tomato purée
1 bay leaf
350ml vegetable stock
260g wholewheat spaghetti
½ bunch basil leaves, torn
Parmesan, to serve (optional)
Sea salt
Freshly ground black pepper

1. Heat the olive oil in a large, heavy-based saucepan, over a low–medium heat. Add the onion, carrots and celery to the pan and gently cook down, stirring often. Cook for 10 minutes until the vegetables have softened.

2. Turn the heat up to medium and add the beef and pork mince and garlic to the pan. Using a wooden spoon, break up the mince as it browns and cooks. It will begin to release a bit of liquid, so continue cooking and stirring until this has evaporated and the meat begins to fry. Browning the meat helps to give the bolognese that wonderful meaty flavour.

3. Once the meat has browned slightly, pour the red wine into the pan and allow to evaporate.

4. Add the passata, tomato purée, bay leaf and stock. Bring to the boil and then reduce to a gentle simmer, cooking for 30 minutes, stirring occasionally to prevent it from sticking. Taste and season with sea salt and black pepper, as desired.

5. Once the sauce has reduced down to a thick consistency with a deep red colour, turn the heat right down and cover with a lid.

6. Cook the pasta in boiling salted water, according to the packet instructions.

7. Drain the pasta and stir through the Bolognese sauce, along with the torn basil. Sprinkle over the grated Parmesan, if using, to serve.

Chicken and Barley Stew

This hearty stew is perfect on a cold day. Pearl barley is full of beneficial nutrients, reduces hunger and is a good source of beta-glucans, which help to lower cholesterol.

SERVES 4

3 skinless, boneless chicken breasts
1 tbsp olive oil
2 celery sticks, finely diced
1 onion, peeled and finely diced
2 carrots, peeled and finely diced
1 large leek, sliced
2 garlic cloves, finely chopped
1 bay leaf
1 tbsp fresh thyme leaves
40g pearl barley
400g baby new potatoes, halved
800ml vegetable stock
Large handful of kale
Sea salt
Freshly ground black pepper

1. Place the chicken in a large saucepan and cover with cold water. Bring to the boil, then turn the heat down slightly and simmer for about 10 minutes until the chicken is cooked through (when it is no longer pink and the juices run clear). Remove from the heat.
2. In a large casserole dish, heat the olive oil over a medium heat and add the onion, carrots and leek. Fry for about 8 minutes until they are beginning to soften, ensuring that they do not colour in the pan.
3. Add the garlic and fry for a further 1–2 minutes. Stir in the bay leaf, thyme, pearl barley and potatoes and season well with sea salt and black pepper.
4. Pour in the stock and bring to the boil, then reduce the heat and simmer for 30–35 minutes until the vegetables, potatoes and pearl barley are tender.
5. Slice or shred the chicken and add to the vegetable stew, along with the kale. Cook for a further 5 minutes and serve.

Carbs 65g	
Calories 420	
Fat 5g	
Protein 40g	

Low-calorie Sunday Dinner

This low-calorie roast dinner recipe is the perfect weekend meal for two. It is low in calories, high in protein and full of delicious veggies. Feel free to double this recipe for more people.

SERVES 2

4 potatoes, peeled and halved
2 skinless, boneless chicken breasts
Low-calorie cooking spray
1 onion, cut into wedges
1 tsp dried Italian herbs
1 leek, finely sliced
2 garlic cloves, finely sliced
2 tbsp reduced-fat soft cheese
Small handful of Cheddar, grated (or your choice of cheese)
500ml chicken stock
1 tsp onion powder
1 tsp garlic powder
2 tsp gravy powder, mixed with 2 tsp water
15g plain flour
40ml milk
1 free-range egg
2 large carrots, sliced lengthways
2 large handfuls spring greens
Sea salt
Freshly ground black pepper

1. Bring a large saucepan of water to the boil. Add the potatoes and cook for 5–8 minutes. Drain and leave in the colander while you get on with the rest.
2. Preheat the oven to 190°C/375°F/Gas 5 and warm a baking tray in the oven. While this is heating, spray the potatoes all over with cooking spray and sprinkle with plenty of sea salt and black pepper. When the baking tray is hot, remove from the oven and add the potatoes. Bake in the oven for 40–45 minutes, turning them every 15 minutes or so to ensure they are golden all over.
3. Place the chicken breasts on a small roasting tray and spray with cooking spray. Season with salt and pepper and add the onion. Sprinkle over the dried Italian herbs, then bake in the oven for 30 minutes until the chicken is cooked through (when it is no longer pink and the juices run clear).
4. Heat some more cooking spray in a saucepan over a medium heat and add the leeks and garlic. Fry until soft, taking care not to let it burn. Add the soft cheese and Cheddar and give everything a good mix. You may want to add a splash of milk if the mixture seems a little too thick. Turn the heat right down and keep warm while you get on with the rest.
5. Place a small saucepan over a medium heat and heat the chicken stock, onion and garlic powders and the gravy powder and water until thickened. Keep over a low heat while you do the next step.
6. To make the Yorkshire puddings, spray two holes in a muffin tin with cooking spray. Pop in the oven to heat.

In a large bowl, whisk together the flour, milk, egg and some sea salt. When smooth, remove the muffin tin from the oven and pour the batter into the two greased holes. Return to the oven for about 15 minutes until fluffed up. Don't open the oven while these are cooking as they will collapse.

7. Boil the carrots in another saucepan of water for about 7–10 minutes, or until cooked but still with a nice bite. Remove with a pair of tongs and add the spring greens. These should only take 3–4 minutes to cook. Arrange everything on a plate and serve.

NOTE: the above timings are just a guide. If cooking times differ, try to keep everything warm while you cook the rest.

Carbs 72g

Calories 568

Fat 18.5g

Protein 25.2g

Creamy Ham and Pea Gnocchi

This is such a simple pasta dish that is guaranteed to impress anyone. Smoky, crispy pancetta, sweet peas and delicious, creamy pasta make this an absolute winner for everyone in the family – even the kids.

SERVES 4
800g fresh gnocchi
Low-calorie cooking spray
200g smoked pancetta, cubed
1 onion, finely chopped
4 garlic cloves, finely chopped
150ml vegetable stock
5 tbsp reduced-fat crème fraîche
200g frozen peas
100g reduced-fat mozzarella ball
Sea salt
Freshly ground black pepper

1. Cook the gnocchi for 2 minutes in boiling salted water (or according to the packet instructions). Once cooked, drain and set aside.

2. While the gnocchi is cooking, heat a large frying pan over a medium heat and spray about five times with the cooking spray.

3. Add the pancetta and fry until beginning to turn golden brown and crisp. Add the onion and fry for 2 minutes, stirring frequently. Add the garlic and fry for another minute.

4. Pour in the stock, crème fraîche and peas and stir in the gnocchi until well coated. Tear in the mozzarella and season with some sea salt and some black pepper.

Carbs 35.1g	
Calories 581	
Fat 23.4g	
Protein 55.8g	

Chicken Milanese with Creamy Courgetti

The Parmesan mixed through the crispy panko breadcrumbs seasons the chicken breast and gives it the crunchiest golden finish. We've paired this with a deliciously light but creamy mushroom sauce and courgetti. Feel free to double this recipe for more people.

SERVES 2

2 boneless, skinless chicken breasts
1½ tbsp olive oil
150g chestnut mushrooms, finely sliced
2 garlic cloves, finely chopped
2 courgettes, spiralised
60g reduced-fat soft cheese
1 tbsp plain flour
2 free-range eggs, beaten
100g panko breadcrumbs
1 tbsp Parmesan, grated
Zest of 1 lemon
½ bunch fresh flat-leaf parsley leaves, to serve (optional)
Sea salt
Freshly ground black pepper

1. Place the chicken breasts in a ziplock bag and, using a rolling pin, bash the chicken to about a 1cm thickness (this will help them to cook evenly in the pan and prevent overcooking). Set aside.
2. In a non-stick frying pan, heat ½ tablespoon of the olive oil over a low heat and add the mushrooms. Cook for 4–5 minutes until softened, then add the garlic and cook for a further minute.
3. Add the courgettes, mix well and cook for 3 minutes until cooked through. Spoon in the soft cheese, along with a splash of water, stirring well until you have a nice, thick, creamy sauce.
4. Meanwhile, grab three plates. Place the flour in the first one and the beaten egg in the second. Mix together the panko breadcrumbs, Parmesan and some sea salt and black pepper in the third bowl.
5. Dip each chicken breast in the flour, then the egg and then the breadcrumbs, ensuring they are fully coated in breadcrumbs.
6. Pour the remaining olive oil into a non-stick frying pan over a medium heat and fry the chicken for about 3–4 minutes on each side until it is cooked through (when it is no longer pink and the juices run clear) and the sides are golden and crispy.
7. Serve on a bed of the creamy mushrooms and courgetti and top with the lemon zest and parsley, if using.

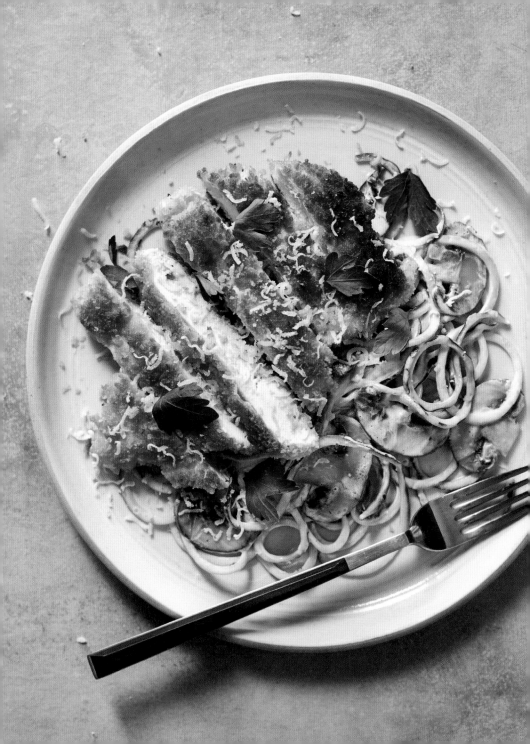

Carbs 52.2g

Calories 468

Fat 10.3g

Protein 41.4g

BBQ Pulled Chicken Burgers

These smoky chicken burgers take no time to rustle up and the low-fat, creamy slaw is the perfect accompaniment to the rich BBQ sauce. Feel free to double this recipe for more people.

SERVES 2

FOR THE PULLED CHICKEN BURGERS
2 boneless, skinless chicken breasts
4 tbsp smoky BBQ sauce
1 tsp chilli sauce
2 brioche buns
Lettuce, to serve

FOR THE SLAW
3 tbsp light mayonnaise
1 tbsp fat-free yoghurt
½ garlic clove, grated
1 carrot, peeled and grated
1 small red onion, finely sliced
¼ white cabbage, grated
4 cherry tomatoes, halved
½ tsp Dijon mustard
1 tsp white wine vinegar
Sea salt
Freshly ground black pepper

1. To make the slaw, simply mix all the ingredients in a large bowl and sprinkle through some sea salt and black pepper to season. You can also add any other grated vegetables you wish. Set aside until needed.
2. Place the chicken breasts in a medium/large saucepan and cover completely with cold water. Bring to the boil.
3. As soon as it is boiling, reduce the heat to a simmer and cook for 12–15 minutes until the breast is cooked through completely (when it is no longer pink and the juices run clear).
4. Remove the chicken from the water and, when hot enough to handle, shred them with two forks.
5. Place the shredded chicken in a bowl and add the BBQ and chilli sauces. Mix well and add some black pepper. Pop on a foil-lined baking tray and place under a hot grill for 2–4 minutes until beginning to caramelise and slightly charring at the edges.
6. Pile the chicken into the brioche buns, topped with the delicious crunchy slaw and lettuce.

Carbs 22.9g

Calories 340

Fat 28.3g

Protein 35.8g

Sweet Potato Cottage Pie

There is something magical about the simplicity of a comforting cottage pie. We've made this one even more nutritious by adding a generous layer of cheesy sweet-potato mash.

SERVES 4

1 tbsp olive oil

500g extra-lean beef mince

1 large onion, finely chopped

1 large carrot, peeled and finely chopped

100g chestnut mushrooms, finely chopped

2 garlic cloves, finely chopped

2 sweet potatoes, peeled and cubed

1 tbsp plain flour

1 tbsp tomato purée

50ml red wine (optional)

400ml beef stock

Skimmed milk, for mashing

Low-fat spread, for mashing

60g reduced-fat Cheddar, grated

Steamed spring greens, to serve

1. Preheat the oven to 200°C/400°F/Gas 6.
2. Heat the oil in a large, non-stick saucepan over a medium heat and brown the mince all over. Remove from the pan.
3. Add the onion, carrot and mushrooms to the same pan and fry for 5 minutes. Stir in the garlic and fry for a further 2 minutes.
4. Cook the chopped sweet potatoes in a pan of boiling water for 8–10 minutes (depending on the size of your cubes) until cooked through.
5. Add the mince to the pan with the vegetables and sprinkle in the plain flour, stirring until combined. Cook for 1 minute.
6. Squeeze in the tomato purée and add the red wine, if using. Reduce slightly before adding the beef stock. Bring to the boil, then reduce the heat and simmer for 15 minutes until thickened.
7. Drain the sweet potatoes and mash with a fork or potato masher, adding small amounts of milk and/or low-fat spread, as desired, to make it creamier.
8. Pour the mince mixture into an ovenproof dish and top with the sweet-potato mash. Add the grated cheese over the top.
9. Bake for 20 minutes until the cheese is golden and melted. Serve with steamed spring greens.

Carbs 11.5g

Calories 392

Fat 23g

Protein 27.6g

Healthier Lasagne

This is the ultimate lasagne recipe, and we've even made it slightly healthier using low-fat crème fraîche instead of a typical white sauce. Summer or winter, this dish is perfect, and can be accompanied by garlic bread or a side salad, depending on what you feel like.

SERVES 6

1 tsp olive oil
500g extra-lean beef mince
1 onion, finely diced
1 celery stick, finely diced
1 carrot, finely diced
3 garlic cloves, finely chopped
1 small glass red wine (optional)
2 tbsp tomato purée
1 tsp Worcestershire sauce
1 tbsp plain flour
1 x 400g tin chopped tomatoes
150ml beef stock (or chicken or vegetable)
1 tsp dried oregano
1 tsp honey
1 bay leaf
9 fresh egg lasagne sheets
200g half-fat crème fraîche
120g reduced-fat mozzarella, grated
50g reduced-fat Cheddar, grated
Sea salt
Freshly ground black pepper

1. Preheat the oven to 200°C/400°F/Gas 6.
2. Heat the olive oil in a large, non-stick pan over a medium–high heat and brown the mince all over for 10 minutes until caramelised and golden. Remove and set aside.
3. Add the onion, celery and carrot to the same pan and fry over a medium heat for 8–10 minutes until softened but not too brown. Stir in the garlic and fry for 2 minutes.
4. Add the red wine and let this bubble down for 3 minutes. Stir in the tomato purée, Worcestershire sauce and plain flour. Cook for 1–2 minutes.
5. Add the chopped tomatoes, stock, oregano, honey and bay leaf. Bring to the boil, then reduce to a simmer and cook for 30–35 minutes until thickened.
6. Pour a layer of the ragu into an ovenproof dish, then cover with a layer of lasagne sheets, followed by more ragu and so forth until you've used up all the lasagne and ragu, finishing with a layer of lasagne sheets.
7. Spread over the crème fraîche and season well with sea salt and black pepper.
8. Sprinkle over the grated cheeses and bake in the oven for 20–25 minutes until bubbling and golden.

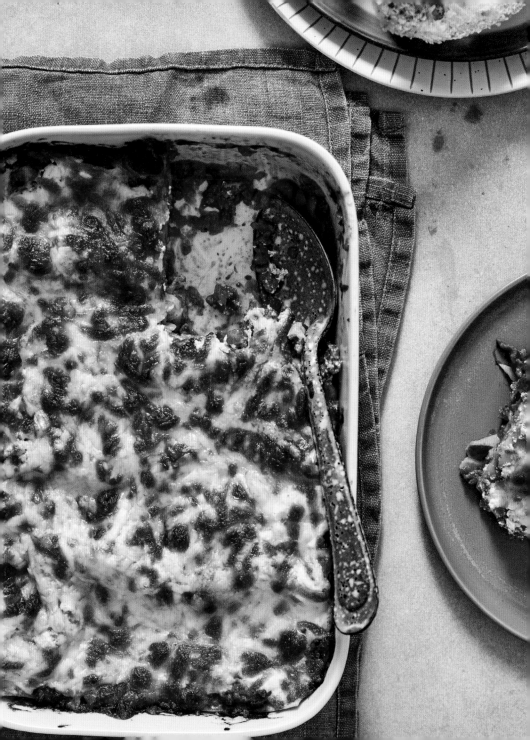

Carbs 70.5g

Calories 563

Fat 18.6g

Protein 25.9g

Pizza Jacket Potato

This nation is obsessed with jacket potatoes. It is also obsessed with pizza. So, why not combine the two? Behold the Pizza Jacket Potato. Feel free to double this recipe for more people.

SERVES 2

2 large baking potatoes, washed and patted dry
3 garlic cloves, finely chopped
Low-calorie cooking spray
6 tbsp passata
½ tsp dried Italian herbs
8 slices pepperoni, sliced into half-moons
70g reduced-fat Cheddar, grated
70g reduced-fat mozzarella, grated
Fresh rocket, to serve
Sea salt
Freshly ground black pepper

1. Preheat the oven to 200°C/400°F/Gas 6 .
2. Prick the potatoes all over with a fork and bake in the oven for 1 hour.
2. Meanwhile, gently fry the garlic in a few sprays of low-calorie cooking spray for 1 minute until softened, then pour in the passata and Italian herbs. Cook over a medium heat until heated through.
3. Stir in the pepperoni and season with salt and black pepper. Keep warm until the potatoes are cooked.
4. Remove the potatoes from the oven, cut a cross in the skin at the top of each one and open them up, taking care not to burn yourself.
5. Spoon over the tomato sauce and top with both the cheeses. Return to the oven and bake until the cheese is golden and melted. Top with some fresh rocket and tuck in!

Carbs 66.5g

Calories 427

Fat 6.3g

Protein 13.5g

Kickin' Penne al'Arrabiata

Give your workout the kick it needs with this spicy tomato pasta. Ready in just 30 minutes, it's the perfect midweek, store-cupboard meal.

SERVES 4

300g penne
1 tbsp olive oil
1 heaped tsp dried chilli flakes
4 garlic cloves, finely chopped
1 tbsp tomato purée
2 × 400g tins chopped tomatoes
1 tsp maple syrup (or runny honey)
125g ball reduced-fat mozzarella, torn into chunks
10 basil leaves, torn
Sea salt
Freshly ground black pepper

1. Add the pasta to a pan of vigorously boiling water and cook according to the packet instructions (it should take about 12 minutes).
2. Meanwhile, heat the olive oil in a large frying pan over a low–medium heat and add the chilli flakes and garlic. Fry for 2 minutes until softened but not browned.
3. Stir through the tomato purée and pour in the chopped tomatoes, along with the maple syrup and a sprinkling of sea salt and black pepper. Stir the sauce well and simmer for 5 minutes.
4. When the pasta is cooked, drain and add to the tomato sauce, tossing until well combined.
5. Serve in bowls, topped with the mozzarella and basil.

TOP TIP: switch the pasta for wholemeal pasta to up your fibre intake.

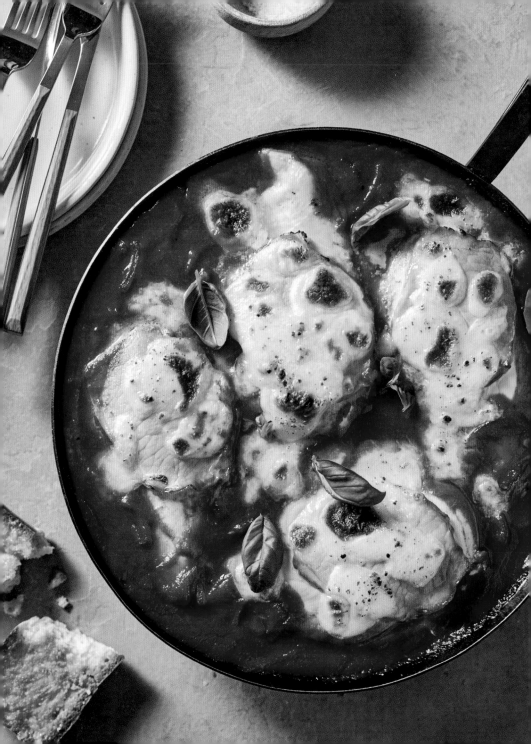

Carbs 43.4g
Calories 457
Fat 7.2g
Protein 53.8g

Hunter's Chicken

An all-time pub classic. Juicy chicken breast, smoky bacon and melted mozzarella, all baked within a delicious smoky tomato sauce.

SERVES 4
Low-calorie cooking spray
1 large red onion, finely sliced
3 garlic cloves, finely chopped
1 tbsp smoked paprika
2 tbsp tomato purée
700g passata
4 tbsp reduced-sugar-and-salt BBQ sauce
1 tsp Worcestershire sauce
2 tsp sugar-free maple syrup
4 reduced-fat smoked bacon medallions
4 boneless, skinless chicken breasts
120g reduced-fat mozzarella, torn into chunks
Large handful of fresh basil leaves
Sea salt
Freshly ground black pepper

FOR THE GARLIC BREAD
2 petit pains, halved lengthways
1 garlic clove
Low-fat spread (optional)

1. Preheat the oven to 180°C/350°F/Gas 4.
2. In a flameproof oven dish, heat around ten sprays of low-calorie cooking spray over a medium heat and, once hot, add the red onion. Fry for 3–5 minutes until softened and lightly golden.
3. Add the garlic and fry for a further minute, stirring. Sprinkle over the smoked paprika and stir, ensuring the onions and garlic are completely coated. Add the tomato purée and stir again.
4. Pour over the passata, BBQ sauce, Worcestershire sauce, maple syrup and 150ml water. Stir well and season with sea salt and lots of black pepper. Bring to a simmer and leave to cook for a couple of minutes.
5. Place the bacon medallions on top of the chicken breasts, so that they lightly wrap them, and nestle them into the sauce.
6. Top with the mozzarella and bake in the oven for about 20 minutes until the chicken is cooked through (when it is no longer pink and the juices run clear).
7. While the chicken is baking, toast your bread and, once ready, slice the top off the garlic clove and rub it all over the toast. Spread with low-fat spread, if desired.
8. When the chicken is cooked, remove from the oven and scatter over the basil leaves. Serve with the garlic bread and enjoy.

Carbs 83.3g

Calories 596

Fat 14.5g

Protein 26.6g

Halloumi and Pea Risotto

This delicious vegetarian dish will have all the meat-eaters jealous. Golden, crisp halloumi sat on top of a rich, green risotto – this really is a crowd-pleaser.

SERVES 4
1 tsp olive oil
1 tsp low-fat spread
1 onion, finely diced
2 garlic cloves, finely diced
350g Arborio (risotto) rice
100ml white wine
750ml vegetable stock
400g frozen peas, defrosted
225g reduced-fat halloumi, cut into thick strips
Zest of 1 lemon
Parmesan, to serve
Sea salt
Freshly ground black pepper

1. Melt the olive oil and low-fat spread in a frying pan over a medium heat. Add the onion and fry for about 3–5 minutes until softened but not golden. Add the garlic to the pan and fry for a further 2 minutes.
2. Add the rice and stir for a minute, then increase the heat and pour in the wine. Cook until the rice has absorbed the liquid.
3. Stir in the stock, a ladleful at a time (adding another one only when the previous one has been completely absorbed) until the stock has been used up and the rice is tender and creamy.
4. When you have used up all of the stock, blitz half the peas in a blender and add to the pan, along with the remaining whole peas. Heat through for a minute or so.
5. Turn the grill to high and grill the halloumi strips for 1–2 minutes on each side until golden.
6. Stir the lemon zest into the risotto and season with sea salt and black pepper.
7. Divide the risotto between bowls and serve with the golden grilled halloumi on top.

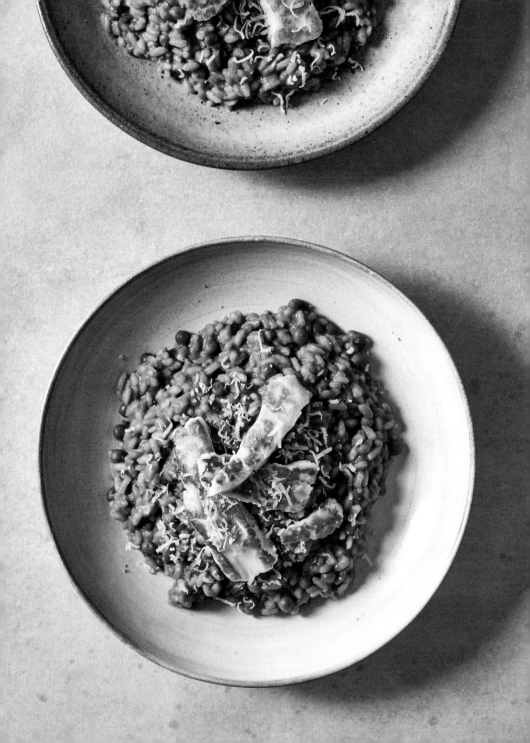

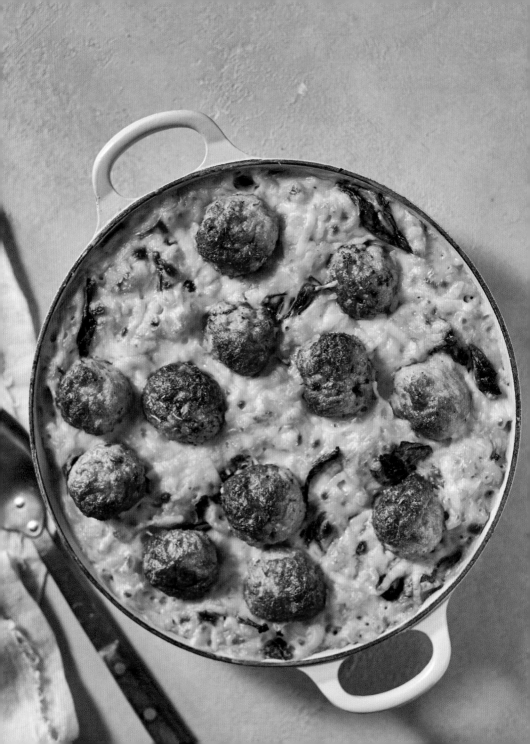

Carbs 40.8g

Calories 465

Fat 12.3g

Protein 47g

Melty Meatball Mac and Cheese

This dish is pure indulgence – but don't worry, I've made it so you don't have to worry about the calories. Did I mention it's full of protein?

SERVES 4

FOR THE MEATBALLS
500g chicken mince
1 garlic clove, grated
1 tsp dried Italian herbs
1 free-range egg, beaten
Low-calorie cooking spray
Sea salt
Freshly ground black
  pepper

**FOR THE MAC AND
CHEESE**
50g low-fat spread
50g plain flour
600ml skimmed milk
300g macaroni
50g reduced-fat Cheddar,
  grated
50g reduced-fat
  mozzarella, grated
1 tsp Dijon mustard
2 large handfuls of fresh
  baby spinach

1. Preheat the oven to 190°C/375°F/Gas 5.
2. To make the meatballs, mix the chicken mince, garlic, dried herbs, egg and a sprinkling of salt and pepper with your hands and form into about twelve balls.
3. Lay the balls on a baking tray, spray with low-calorie cooking spray and pop in the oven for 15 minutes until almost cooked through.
4. Meanwhile, boil the pasta in salted water for about 8–10 minutes, or until al dente.
5. While the meatballs and pasta are cooking, make the sauce. Melt the low-fat spread in a saucepan over a medium heat and, once melted, stir in the flour. Cook, stirring, for 1–2 minutes.
6. Slowly pour in the milk, whisking constantly. Once all the milk has been added, keep whisking over a medium heat until thickened, then add the grated cheeses, Dijon mustard and fresh spinach. Stir well and season with black pepper.
7. Once the pasta is cooked, drain and mix through the cheese sauce. Place the mixture in an ovenproof dish and top with the meatballs.
8. Bake for 15–20 minutes until the chicken meatballs are completely cooked through and the mac and cheese is golden and bubbling.

Carbs 2.7g	
Calories 238	
Fat 12.8g	
Protein 27.2g	

Lighter Ham and Leek Quiche

This recipe is perfect for lunch or a picnic. Switch up the filling ingredients to suit your taste; it's so incredibly versatile, and because it is crustless, it comes in at a fraction of the calories.

SERVES 4

Low-calorie cooking spray
150g leeks, finely sliced
5 large eggs, beaten
120g fat-free quark
¼ tsp garlic granules
150g cooked ham, sliced into long, thick matchsticks
3 spring onions, finely sliced
100g reduced-fat Cheddar, grated
Sea salt
Freshly ground black pepper

1. Preheat the oven to 180°C/350°F/ Gas 4.
2. In a frying pan, heat about ten sprays of cooking spray over a medium heat and fry the leeks for 5–7 minutes until softened. Set aside to cool slightly.
3. Meanwhile, place the eggs and quark in a large bowl and whisk until combined and smooth. Season with sea salt, black pepper and the garlic granules.
4. Add the ham and leeks to the bowl, along with the spring onions. Add three-quarters of the cheese, giving everything a stir.
5. Grease a round tart tin (about 22cm) with cooking spray, rubbing around the edges with your fingers.
6. Pour the mixture into the tin and scatter the remaining cheese on top. Bake in the oven for 20–25 minutes until the mixture is beginning to turn golden. If you prefer it a little more golden, simply pop under a hot grill for 2–3 minutes to finish.

Slow-cooker Chicken and Chorizo Casserole

This really is comfort food at its finest. Think wholesome chicken stew – Spanish style! Just pop everything in the slow cooker in the morning and by late afternoon, it's ready.

SERVES 4

200g chorizo, cut into large chunks

4 boneless, skinless chicken thighs

2 onions, cut into wedges

2 red peppers, deseeded and sliced into large chunks

500g baby new potatoes, halved

4 garlic cloves, finely chopped

1 × 400g tin butter beans, drained and rinsed

1 × 400g tin chopped tomatoes

6 sundried tomatoes

250ml chicken stock

1 tbsp tomato purée

2 tsp smoked paprika

10 black olives

½ tsp dried chilli flakes

1 tsp honey

Zest of ½ lemon

Sea salt

Freshly ground black pepper

Green, leafy vegetables, to serve

1. Place all the ingredients in a slow cooker and cook either on high for 4½ hours or on low for 8 hours until the chicken is cooked (when it is no longer pink and the juices run clear) and the vegetables are tender.
2. Serve with your favourite green, leafy vegetables.

Carbs 51g

Calories 431

Fat 8.4g

Protein 38.5g

Slow-Cooker Moroccan Lamb Tagine

This authentic Moroccan slow-cooker lamb tagine combines just the right variety of spices to bring you a rich, warming crowd-pleaser.

SERVES 4

600g lean lamb, diced
1 tbsp olive oil
1 cinnamon stick, snapped in two
1 tsp ground ginger
1 tsp ground cumin
1 tsp ground coriander
½ tsp ground turmeric
1 × 400g tin chickpeas, drained and rinsed
1 large onion, roughly chopped
2 carrots, roughly chopped
1 aubergine, cut into 3cm chunks
3 garlic cloves, peeled and finely chopped
1 tbsp maple syrup
80g dried apricots
600ml lamb stock (or chicken stock)
200g couscous
200ml boiling water
Sea salt
Freshly ground black pepper
Freshly chopped parsley, to garnish (optional)

1. Set the slow cooker to high for 20 minutes, while you prepare your ingredients.
2. Turn the slow cooker to low and add the lamb, along with the olive oil, cinnamon and ground spices. Season well with sea salt and black pepper. Use a spoon to mix all the spices to coat the lamb.
3. Add the remaining ingredients (apart from the couscous and boiling water) and pop the lid on. Cook on low for 8–10 hours until the lamb is tender and the vegetables are cooked.
4. About 10 minutes before you are ready to serve, place the couscous in a large bowl, cover with the boiling water and then cover the bowl tightly with cling film. Leave for 5–10 minutes until all the water has been absorbed and the couscous is soft. Fluff with a fork before serving, then spoon the tagine over the top.

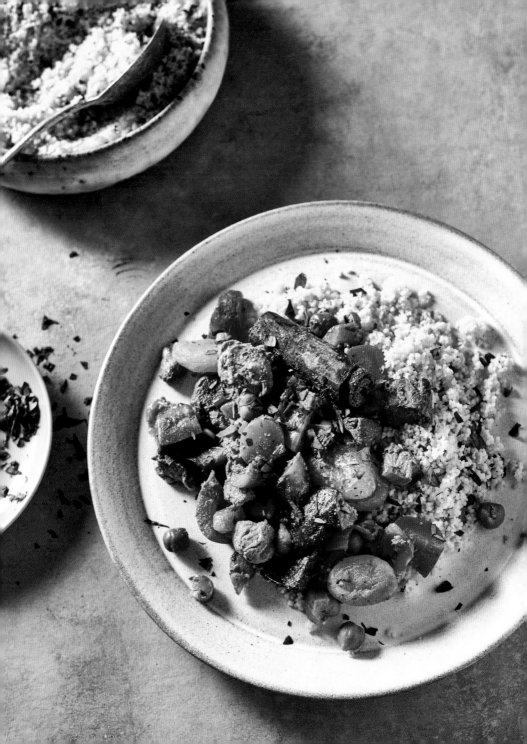

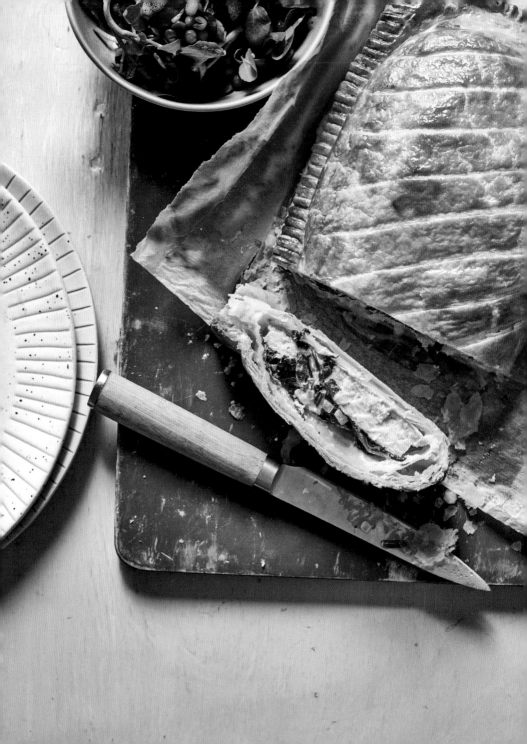

Carbs 31g	
Calories 496	
Fat 24.4g	
Protein 36.4g	

Salmon Wellington

We all love a Wellington and this one is no exception. It is lighter than a normal beef Wellington and much easier to make. I think you're going to love it.

SERVES 5

FOR THE SALMON WELLINGTON
1 tsp olive oil
1 tsp low-fat spread
2 small onions, finely chopped
2 garlic cloves, finely chopped
220g baby spinach
180g reduced-fat soft cheese
1 tbsp capers, lightly chopped
Zest of ½ lemon
1 half-side of salmon (available in most supermarkets)
1 packet ready-rolled light puff pastry
1 free-range egg, beaten
Sea salt
Freshly ground black pepper

FOR THE WATERCRESS AND PEA SALAD
200g frozen peas
1 tbsp white wine vinegar
1 tbsp olive oil
1 tsp Dijon mustard
80g watercress

1. Preheat the oven to 190°C/375°F/Gas 5.
2. In a large frying pan, heat the olive oil and low-fat spread over a medium heat and fry the onions for about 5–7 minutes until soft. Stir in the garlic and fry for a further 2 minutes.
3. Add the spinach, stirring well as it wilts. Once wilted, season well with sea salt and black pepper and remove from the heat.
4. Leave the spinach to cool to room temperature, then stir in the soft cheese, capers and lemon zest.
5. Lay out the puff pastry sheet so it is vertical in front of you. Brush around the edges with a little beaten egg.
6. Place the salmon on the nearest end to you, score four lines through the top of it (not too deep) and spoon over the cheesy spinach sauce.
7. Pull the farthest end of pastry over the top of the salmon and use a fork to press down the sides (you may need to cut off some excess).
8. Brush the top of the pastry with extra egg and bake in the oven for 35–40 minutes until the pastry is crisp and golden and the salmon is cooked through.
9. Meanwhile, boil the peas for 3 minutes and then drain.
10. In a large bowl, mix together the white wine vinegar, olive oil and Dijon mustard. Add the cooked peas and watercress and mix through.
11. Slice the salmon Wellington into five pieces and serve with the pea salad.

TRAYBAKES AND ONE PAN

Carbs 37.7g

Calories 560

Fat 20g

Protein 48.7g

Peri Peri Chicken and Chorizo Traybake

I think that this one-pan traybake will become a firm favourite in your house – it's smoky, sweet, spicy and full to the brim with flavour.

SERVES 4

8 chicken drumsticks
225g ring chorizo, sliced into chunks
2 corn-on-the-cobs, halved
700g baby new potatoes, quartered
2 red peppers, deseeded and cut into thick wedges
1 large onion, cut into large wedges
2 garlic cloves, unpeeled
25g peri peri seasoning
1 tbsp smoked paprika
1 tbsp olive oil
1 tbsp sugar-free maple syrup
1 tbsp tomato purée
3 spring onions, finely sliced
Sea salt
Freshly ground black pepper

1. Preheat the oven to 190°C/375°F/Gas 5.
2. Place the chicken, chorizo, corn, new potatoes, red peppers, onion and garlic in a large roasting tray.
3. In a small bowl, mix together the peri peri seasoning, smoked paprika, olive oil, maple syrup, tomato purée, sea salt and black pepper to form a loose paste, adding more oil if it seems a little thick.
4. Pour over the other ingredients in the roasting tray and rub all around until everything is well combined.
5. Bake in the oven for 1 hour until the chicken is cooked through (when it is no longer pink and the juices run clear). Give everything a good toss after 30 minutes, ensuring that you flip the drumsticks over.
6. Serve with the spring onions scattered over the top.

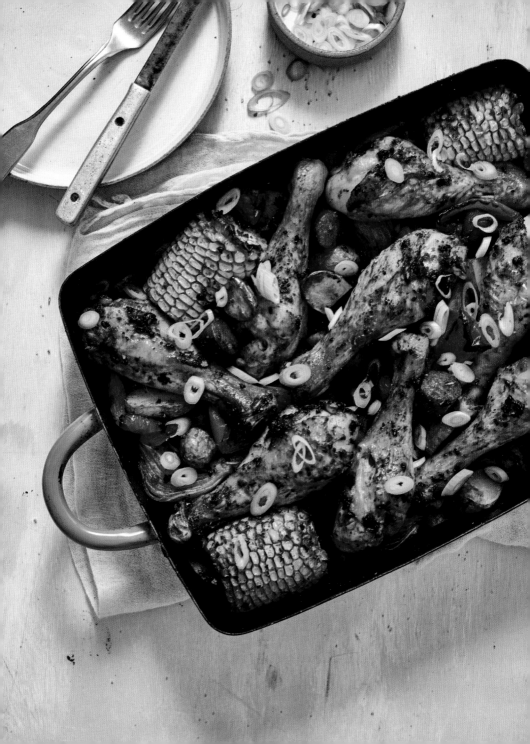

Carbs 36.1g

Calories 385

Fat 10.8g

Protein 33g

Tikka Cod Traybake

Think of this dish as the easiest curry you'll ever make. Cod is a great source of protein and is very low in calories. It is also a great source of phosphorous – a mineral needed to maintain strong bones and a healthy body. You could, however, use pollock or salmon in this dish, instead.

SERVES 4

6 tbsp tikka paste (or tikka spice marinade)

500g baby potatoes, quartered

2 red peppers, deseeded and sliced

2 onions, sliced into wedges

10 cherry tomatoes, halved

1 tbsp olive oil

1 × 400g tin chickpeas, drained and rinsed

4 sustainable cod fillets

5 spring onions, finely sliced

½ bunch fresh coriander

½ bunch fresh mint leaves

Sea salt

Freshly ground black pepper

1. Preheat the oven to 200°C/400°F/Gas 6. Line a large baking tray with non-stick baking paper.

2. In a large bowl, mix 4 tablespoons of the tikka paste with the potatoes, ensuring they are nicely coated.

3. Transfer to the lined baking tray, along with the peppers, onions and cherry tomatoes. Drizzle with the olive oil and season with sea salt and freshly ground black pepper. Mix everything together.

4. Bake for 20–25 minutes until the potatoes are beginning to turn golden and soft. Remove from the oven and stir through the chickpeas.

5. Place the cod fillets on top of the vegetables, potatoes and chickpeas, then spoon over the remaining tikka paste and return to the oven for a further 10 minutes until the cod is cooked and flakes easily.

6. Serve with the spring onions, coriander and mint sprinkled over.

Carbs 10.2g

Calories 309

Fat 18g

Protein 25.1g

Sweet Chilli Salmon Traybake

This is one of my favourite traybakes ever – you won't be able to get enough of the delicious glaze, which goes perfectly with the roasted salmon.

SERVES 4

30g fresh ginger, grated
4 garlic cloves, grated
2 red chillies, deseeded, then 1 finely chopped and 1 finely sliced
2 tbsp white wine vinegar
3 tbsp low-sodium soy sauce
1 tbsp maple syrup (or runny honey)
½ red onion, finely chopped
4 skinless salmon fillets
300g tenderstem broccoli
100g asparagus
Low-calorie cooking spray
½ bunch fresh coriander leaves
2 tsp sesame seeds
Juice of 1 lime
½ bunch spring onions, finely sliced

1. Preheat the oven to 190°C/375°F/Gas 5.
2. In a small bowl, mix together the ginger, garlic, chopped chilli (keep the sliced one for a garnish), vinegar, soy sauce, maple syrup and red onion. Set aside until needed.
3. Place the salmon fillets in a large baking tray and nestle the broccoli and asparagus around them. Pour over the glaze and spray the vegetables and salmon about five times with low-calorie cooking spray.
4. Cover tightly with foil and roast for 20 minutes until the salmon is cooked and the vegetables are tender.
5. Remove from the oven and top with the fresh coriander, sesame seeds and lime juice. Scatter over the spring onions and sliced chilli and serve.

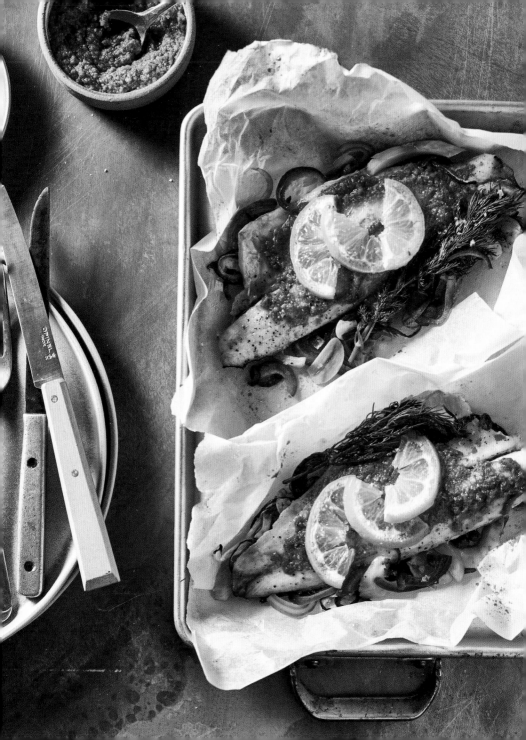

Carbs 17.8g

Calories 248

Fat 7.6g

Protein 27.2g

Easy Sea Bass Parcels

This is the quickest and easiest way to cook fish (in my opinion). You can pop everything in some baking paper, wrap it up, pop it in the oven and get on with a workout. Your food will be done in no time.

SERVES 2

8 cherry tomatoes
1 red onion, finely sliced
1 fennel bulb, finely sliced
2 garlic cloves, finely sliced
2 tsp capers
Small handful of fresh dill (or use fresh basil leaves)
2 sea bass fillets (or use cod/trout/bream)
2 tsp olive oil
2 heaped tsp red pesto
1 lemon, cut into slices
2 tbsp white wine (optional, but works great)
Sea salt
Freshly ground black pepper

1. Preheat the oven to 190°C/375°F/Gas 5.
2. Grab some non-stick baking paper (or foil) and cut two squares large enough to encase the fish and the vegetables in two parcels – about 40 × 40cm each should do the trick.
3. Divide the vegetables between the two squares, then add the garlic, capers and dill (or basil) and pop the fish on top. Season well with sea salt and black pepper and drizzle with the olive oil. At this stage, you could also add any additional flavours you might like, such as chilli flakes or different herbs.
4. Spread the pesto over the fish and place the lemon slices on top. Spoon over the wine, if using.
5. Pull the sides of the paper up and wrap the fish tightly, making sure that it's completely enclosed (the secret to this recipe is to ensure there is nowhere for the steam to escape, as it is this that will cook the fish and vegetables).
6. Bake the parcels for 15–20 minutes until the fish is cooked and the vegetables are tender but still have a nice crunch.

Carbs 35.6g

Calories 272

Fat 9.2g

Protein 11.8g

Magic Pasta

This type of pasta cooking has taken the social media world by storm. The sauce is made using the vegetables and the pasta water, so you literally just need one large frying pan (this needs to be straight/high-sided) – then pop everything in and watch a delicious pasta dish develop in no time. It really is magic!

SERVES 4

300g spaghetti

400g cherry tomatoes (try to get different coloured tomatoes if you can)

Zest of 1 large lemon

1 tbsp extra virgin olive oil

1 tsp chilli flakes

2 garlic cloves, finely sliced

300g curly kale

1 litre boiling water

70g Parmesan, grated

½ bunch fresh basil leaves, torn

Sea salt

Freshly ground black pepper

1. Place all the ingredients, except the kale, Parmesan and basil, in a large, high-sided pan.
2. Bring to the boil over a high heat and, once boiling, set a timer for 9–10 minutes. Use a pair of tongs or a large fork to stir the pasta frequently until it is al dente and has absorbed most of the water. For the last 3 minutes, add the kale and stir through.
3. Stir in the Parmesan and serve with the fresh basil.

Carbs 17.9g

Calories 453

Fat 18.9g

Protein 53.3g

One-pan Caprese Chicken

This delicious chicken dish covered in melting mozzarella will make anyone go back for more. The rich tomato sauce and creamy mozzarella deliver a real taste sensation, plus it only uses one pan, so less washing up and more time for workouts!

SERVES 2

1 tbsp olive oil

2 boneless, skinless chicken breasts

1 small red onion, finely chopped

3 garlic cloves, finely sliced

200g tinned chopped tomatoes

200g mixed colour cherry tomatoes, halved

10 pitted green olives

1 tbsp balsamic vinegar

1 tbsp maple syrup

200g light mozzarella ball

Sea salt

Freshly ground black pepper

TO SERVE

Large handful of rocket leaves

2 crusty bread rolls

1. Preheat the grill to high.
2. Put the olive oil in a medium-sized, ovenproof frying pan (or cast-iron skillet) over a medium–high heat and add the chicken breasts. Fry for 2–3 minutes on each side until golden brown.
3. Add the onion and garlic to the pan and fry for another minute. Add the tomatoes, olives, balsamic vinegar and maple syrup and season well with sea salt and black pepper.
4. Tear the mozzarella into large pieces and dot around the pan. Place the pan under the grill for 10 minutes until the chicken is cooked through (when it is no longer pink and the juices run clear).
5. Serve with a large handful of rocket leaves scattered over the top and a crusty roll each.

Carbs 61g	
Calories 441	
Fat 12.2g	
Protein 21.5g	

Sticky Sausage and Red Onion Traybake

Think sausage casserole, but easier. This traybake is earthy with sweet potato, carrots, garlic and caramelised red onion, mixed together with roasted sausages, a sticky syrup and a delicious wholegrain mustard glaze.

SERVES 4

2 tbsp balsamic vinegar
2 tbsp maple syrup
1 tbsp wholegrain mustard
600g sweet potatoes, cut into 2cm chunks
350g red pepper, deseeded and thickly sliced
400g red onion, cut into thick wedges
2 carrots, peeled and cut into 2cm chunks
4 garlic cloves, crushed
8 reduced-fat pork sausages
1 tbsp olive oil
1 tbsp dried thyme
1 tbsp fennel seeds

1. Preheat the oven to 190°C/375°F/Gas 5.
2. In a small bowl, mix together the balsamic vinegar, maple syrup and wholegrain mustard. Set aside.
3. Put the sweet potato, red pepper, red onion, carrots and garlic in a large baking tray.
4. Add the sausages and drizzle over the olive oil, mixing well to ensure everything is well oiled. Sprinkle over the dried thyme and fennel seeds.
5. Bake in the oven for 35 minutes, then remove and pour over the syrupy glaze you made at the beginning. Pop back in the oven for a further 10 minutes, or until the sweet potato is cooked through.

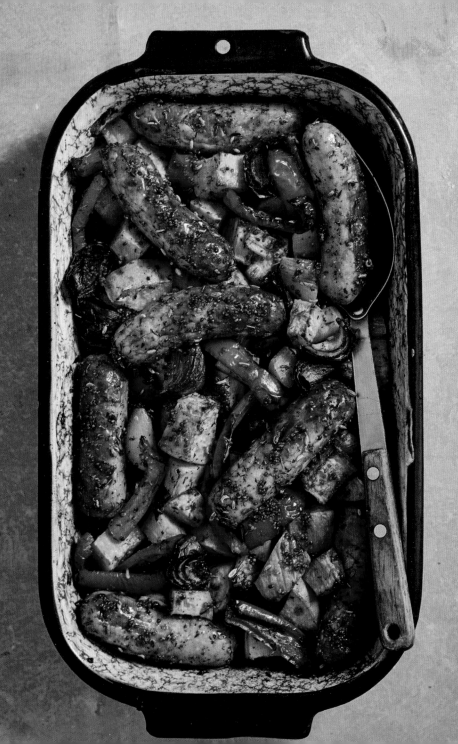

Carbs 30.5g

Calories 382

Fat 13.3g

Protein 33.4g

Teriyaki Chilli Chicken Traybake

I think this one-pan traybake will become a firm favourite in your house – it's smoky, sweet, spicy and full to the brim with flavour!

SERVES 4

1 tbsp olive oil
5 tbsp teriyaki sauce
1 tbsp red wine vinegar
3 garlic cloves, finely grated
Thumb-sized piece of fresh ginger, finely grated
1 tbsp Chinese five-spice powder
8 boneless, skinless chicken thigh fillets
1 bunch spring onions, half left whole and half finely sliced
1 red onion, sliced
250g pak choi (halved lengthways)
120g tenderstem broccoli
150g sugar snap peas
Juice of 1 lime
2 pouches microwave basmati rice
1 tsp dried chilli flakes

1. Preheat the oven to 190°C/375°F/Gas 5.
2. In a small bowl, mix together the olive oil, teriyaki sauce, red wine vinegar, garlic and ginger.
3. Rub the five-spice all over the chicken thighs.
4. Place the whole spring onions and red onion in a large baking tray and add the chicken on top. Spread over the teriyaki glaze, mixing to coat the chicken and the vegetables.
5. Bake for 30 minutes in the preheated oven. Remove from the oven and add the pak choi, broccoli and sugar snap peas with a splash of water and the lime juice. Cover the tray tightly with foil and return to the oven for 10 minutes until the chicken is cooked (when it is no longer pink and the juices run clear).
6. Heat the rice in the microwave according to the packet instructions.
7. Serve the traybake with the finely sliced spring onions and chilli flakes scattered over the top, together with the rice.

Carbs 23.8g

Calories 277

Fat 12.6g

Protein 17.2g

Thai King Prawn Traybake

Prawns don't take long to cook at all – so they only go in for the final five minutes, and the oven does all the rest. I love the spicy Thai coconut flavours here. This one's a winner!

SERVES 4

1 cauliflower, cut
into florets
2 small red onions, peeled
and cut into wedges
1 sweet potato, scrubbed
and cut into 2cm chunks
2 tbsp Thai red curry
paste
1 tsp olive oil
1 × 400g tin light coconut
milk
Juice of 1 lime
½ tsp fish sauce
200g asparagus tips
130g baby corn
250g raw king prawns
½ bunch fresh coriander
1 red chilli, deseeded and
sliced
2 tbsp peanuts, roughly
chopped

1. Preheat the oven to 190°C/375°F/Gas 5.
2. Place the cauliflower, red onions and sweet potato in a large roasting tray and stir in the red curry paste and olive oil until well coated. Bake for 35–40 minutes.
3. Remove from the oven, stir through the coconut milk, lime juice, fish sauce, asparagus, baby corn and prawns.
4. Return to the oven for 5 minutes until the prawns are pink throughout and the vegetables are tender.
5. Serve with the fresh coriander, chilli and peanuts sprinkled over the top.

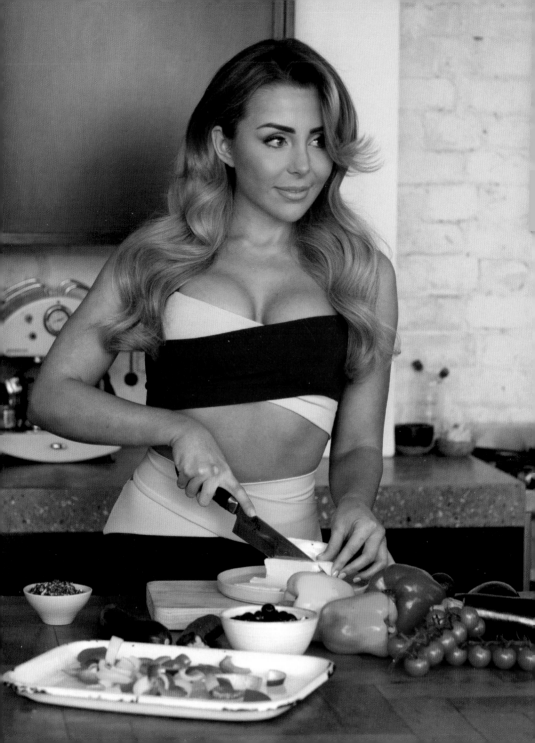

Carbs 17.1g

Calories 428

Fat 26.5g

Protein 28.8g

Mediterranean Halloumi Traybake

Fresh roasted vegetables, salty halloumi and zingy lemon come together here to create a filling vegetarian traybake with little effort required. Simply finish under the grill for delicious crispy, gooey halloumi.

SERVES 4

400g aubergine, cut into 3cm chunks
250g red onion, sliced
270g cherry tomatoes
250g courgettes, thickly sliced
250g mixed colour peppers (we used yellow, orange and red), deseeded and sliced
50g pitted black olives
1 lemon, cut into wedges
1 tbsp olive oil
1 tbsp red wine vinegar
2 tbsp green pesto
400g reduced-fat halloumi, sliced
½ bunch basil
Sea salt
Freshly ground black pepper

1. Preheat the oven to 190°C/375°F/Gas 5.
2. Place all the vegetables in a large baking tray with the olives, lemon wedges, olive oil and red wine vinegar. Stir to combine and season well with salt and pepper.
3. Bake for 30 minutes until the vegetables are tender.
4. Mix through the pesto and lay the slices of halloumi on top. Pop under a hot grill for 3–5 minutes until the halloumi is golden and beginning to crisp.
5. Serve with the basil leaves scattered over the top.

VEGETARIAN AND VEGAN

Carbs 59.1g

Calories 410

Fat 11.9g

Protein 14.3g

Vegan Falafel Flatbreads

These Middle-Eastern falafel flatbreads are perfect for a work-from-home lunch, on-the-go lunch or simply a delicious picnic to enjoy with friends.

MAKES 4

FOR THE FLATBREADS
200g plain flour, plus extra for kneading and rolling
1½ tsp ground coriander
1 tsp sea salt
100ml warm water
1 tbsp olive oil
Low-calorie cooking spray

FOR THE FALAFEL
1 tsp olive oil
1 small onion, finely chopped
2 garlic cloves, grated
1 × 400g tin chickpeas, drained and rinsed
1 tsp ground cumin
1 tsp ground coriander
15g mix of fresh parsley and coriander, roughly chopped
Juice of ¼ lemon
½ tsp salt
25g plain flour

TO SERVE
200g reduced-fat hummus
Shredded lettuce
Halved cherry tomatoes
Finely sliced red onion

1. Preheat the oven to 220°C/425°F/Gas 7. Line a baking tray with non-stick baking paper.
2. To make the dough, combine the flour, ground coriander and salt in a mixing bowl and slowly add the water, little by little, mixing together. Add the oil and knead until you have a smooth, soft dough. If it is too dry, add a splash more water and knead again. Once the dough has come together, tip it out on to a lightly floured surface and knead for 5 minutes. Set the dough aside to rest in a clean bowl while you make the falafel.
3. Heat the oil in a pan and gently fry the onion and garlic for 6–8 minutes, or until soft. Transfer to a food processor with the remaining ingredients and blitz until the mixture has a rough texture but still binds together.
4. Divide into eight balls and slightly squash down. Place on the lined baking tray and bake for 20–25 minutes until crisp and golden.
5. Divide the flatbread dough into four balls. On a clean, lightly floured surface, flatten the balls out into circles using a rolling pin. Add a little more flour to the top (to ensure they don't stick), then flip them and roll out to the thickness of a pound coin.
6. Heat a frying pan over a medium heat and lightly oil with low-calorie cooking spray. Cook each flatbread for 1 minute on each side until puffed up and golden.
7. Cut the falafels in half. Smother hummus over the flatbreads and top with falafel halves, lettuce, cherry tomatoes and red onion, then fold over and serve.

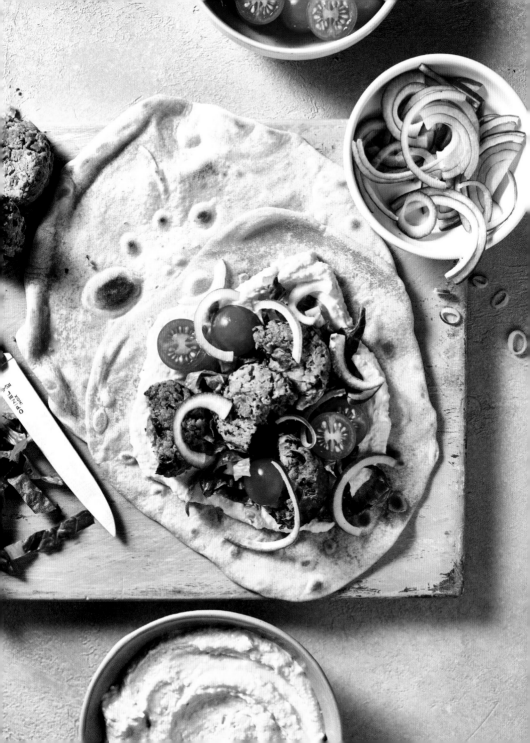

Carbs 67.7g

Calories 329

Fat 2.1g

Protein 7.4g

Easy Mushroom Risotto

Making a good risotto can be a time-consuming task. That's why I have made a really simple yet delicious one that will have your friends and family believe you've taken cooking lessons! It really is so easy. Use whichever mushrooms you like, but I like chestnut and shiitake.

SERVES 4

Low-calorie cooking spray
1 onion, finely chopped
3 garlic cloves, finely chopped
250g mushrooms, finely sliced (I used 125g chestnut and 125g shiitake)
1 tsp dried thyme
2 tbsp red wine vinegar
350g risotto (Arborio) rice
1.2 litres vegetable stock
Zest of ½ lemon
2 tbsp freshly grated Parmesan
1 tbsp finely chopped fresh flat-leaf parsley
Sea salt
Freshly ground black pepper

1. Spray a large, non-stick frying pan about five to eight times with the cooking spray and gently fry the onion and garlic over a low–medium heat.
2. Once softened, add 200g of the mushrooms and continue to cook for 5 minutes, stirring frequently.
3. Add the dried thyme and vinegar, along with the rice. Allow the vinegar to reduce slightly and then add the stock and the remaining mushrooms. Cook over a medium heat for 35–40 minutes until the rice is cooked through but still has a bite. Ensure you are stirring frequently at this point. Season with sea salt and black pepper.
4. Once the rice is cooked to your liking, stir through the lemon zest and half the Parmesan.
5. Finish by scattering over the parsley leaves and the remaining Parmesan.

Carbs 47.1g

Calories 543

Fat 20.2g

Protein 34.7g

Chili 'Non' Carne

This vegan chili 'non' carne is the ultimate comfort food – and you really won't miss the meat. You can use whichever brand of vegan mince you prefer, as long as you brown it nicely in the pan at the start.

SERVES 4

1 tbsp olive oil
500g vegan 'mince'
2 red onions, finely
    chopped
2 celery sticks, finely
    chopped
4 garlic cloves, finely
    chopped
2 tsp ground cumin
1 tsp ground coriander
½ tsp ground cinnamon
1 tsp hot chilli powder
1 tbsp plain flour
1 tbsp tomato purée
300ml vegetable stock
1 × 400g tin chickpeas,
    drained and rinsed
1 × 400g tin kidney beans,
    drained and rinsed
1 × 400g tin chopped
    tomatoes
1 tsp maple syrup
250g brown rice, rinsed
Sea salt
Freshly ground black
    pepper

TO SERVE

Fresh coriander leaves
3 spring onions, finely
    sliced

1. Place a large non-stick frying pan over a medium heat and add the olive oil. Fry the vegan mince for 5 minutes, stirring frequently, until browned all over. Transfer to a bowl and set aside.
2. Add the onions and celery to the pan and fry for a further 3–5 minutes until softened. Stir in the garlic and fry for a further 1–2 minutes until fragrant.
3. Stir in the ground spices and plain flour. Keep stirring and cook for 1 minute.
4. Stir in the tomato purée and then slowly add the vegetable stock, a little at a time, until you have a thickish sauce.
5. Return the mince to the pan, then add the chickpeas, kidney beans, chopped tomatoes and maple syrup. Reduce the heat to medium–low, partially cover the pan with a lid and simmer for 30–35 minutes until the chili has thickened. Season to taste with sea salt and black pepper.
6. Pour the rice into a saucepan, cover with 500ml water and bring to a vigorous boil. As soon as it begins boiling, reduce the heat to low and gently simmer for 30 minutes.
7. After 30 minutes, turn the heat off and cover the pan with a lid for a further 5–10 minutes until any remaining liquid has been absorbed.
8. Serve the rice with the chili spooned over. Sprinkle over the coriander leaves and spring onions.

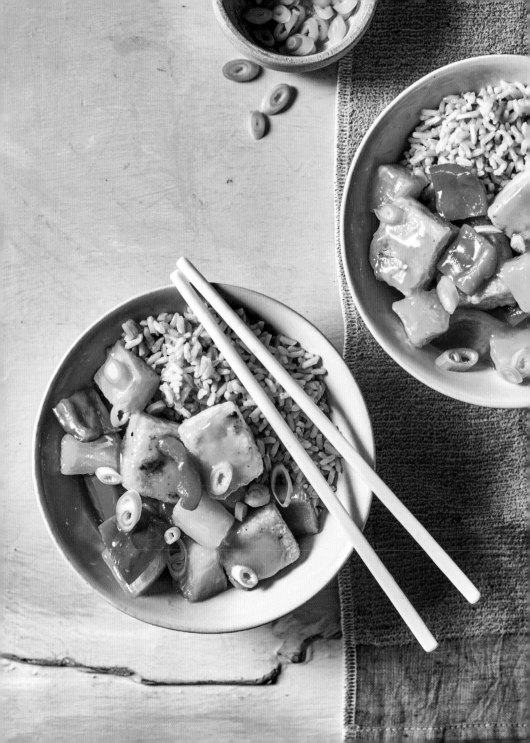

Carbs 50.8g

Calories 373

Fat 11.1g

Protein 12.9g

Vegan Sticky Sweet and Sour Tofu

The juice from the pineapple makes for the perfect sticky, sweet sauce. Paired with the sour vinegar, this makes for a delicious, healthy fakeaway.

SERVES 4
250g brown rice
450g block firm tofu
1 × 432g tin pineapple
chunks in juice, drained
and juice reserved
3 tbsp reduced-sugar
tomato ketchup
2½ tbsp rice wine vinegar
1 tbsp low-sodium
soy sauce
1 tbsp maple syrup
2 tbsp cornflour
1 tbsp olive oil
1 red pepper, deseeded
and cut into small
chunks
1 green pepper, deseeded
and cut into small
chunks
2 garlic cloves, finely
chopped
Sea salt
Freshly ground black
pepper

1. Place the rice in a large saucepan. Pour over 500ml water and bring to a vigorous boil over a high heat. As soon as it begins to boil, reduce the heat to low and gently simmer for 30 minutes.
2. Turn the heat off and cover the pan with a lid for about 5–10 minutes until any remaining liquid has been absorbed by the rice.
3. Drain the tofu, then lay on a sheet of kitchen paper with a second piece on top. Weigh this down, using a heavy book or pot and allow the excess water to slowly drain out. This can be done for anything from an hour to overnight, if left in the fridge. Set aside, while you get on with the sauce.
4. Combine the pineapple juice, ketchup, vinegar, soy sauce and maple syrup in a small saucepan and bring to a simmer over a medium heat, whisking to combine. Mix 1 tablespoon of the cornflour with a splash of water, then add to the sauce and whisk until thickened.
5. Place the remaining cornflour in a bowl and season with a little salt and pepper. Pat the tofu dry, cut into bite-sized cubes and toss in the seasoned cornflour until lightly coated.
6. Heat the oil in a frying pan over a medium–high heat and fry the tofu for about 4–5 minutes until golden. Remove and set aside. Add the peppers and garlic to the pan and stir-fry until slightly softened.
7. Add the pineapple, sauce and tofu to the pan. Reduce the heat to medium and cook, stirring often, until the tofu and pineapple are hot. Serve with the brown rice when ready.

Carbs 37.9g

Calories 249

Fat 4.7g

Protein 11.3g

Leftover Egg-fried Rice

I love the simplicity of this vegetarian dish, but if you want to add some chicken breast, prawns or lean beef, be my guest.

SERVES 4
Low-calorie cooking spray
1 onion, finely diced
1 red pepper, deseeded and finely diced
½ courgette, finely diced
2 garlic cloves, finely chopped
1 tsp Chinese five-spice
350g leftover cooked long-grain rice, cooled
250g frozen peas
3 large free-range eggs, beaten
2 tbsp low-sodium soy sauce
½ bunch spring onions, finely sliced
Sriracha, for drizzling
Sea salt
Freshly ground black pepper

1. In a large, non-stick frying pan (or wok), heat about 10–15 sprays of low-calorie cooking spray over a high heat, then stir-fry the onion, red pepper and courgette for 2 minutes until softened, stirring constantly.
2. Throw in the garlic and five-spice and stir well. Add the cooked rice and fry for a further 3–4 minutes, stirring constantly.
3. Add the peas and stir-fry for 2 minutes. Add the beaten eggs and stir-fry for another 2 minutes, making sure to break up the eggs as they scramble.
4. Add the soy sauce and season with a sprinkling of sea salt and some black pepper.
5. Once the eggs have set and the rice is piping hot, add the spring onions and drizzle with hot and sweet sriracha.

Carbs 71.1g

Calories 593

Fat 27.3g

Protein 20.5g

Vegan Carbonara

You wouldn't believe how creamy a sauce can be made with cashews and this pairs perfectly with meaty mushrooms and sweet garlic. Who said vegan food was boring?

SERVES 2

85g cashew nuts
150g spaghetti
100ml unsweetened
  almond milk
¼ tsp dried oregano
¼ tsp smoked paprika
1 tbsp olive oil
200g chestnut
  mushrooms, finely
  sliced
4 garlic cloves, finely
  chopped
2 tbsp vegan Parmesan,
  grated, to serve
¼ bunch fresh flat leaf
  parsley (optional)
Sea salt
Freshly ground black
  pepper

1. Soak the cashew nuts in very hot water (but not boiling) for 15 minutes. Set aside.
2. Cook the spaghetti in a pan of salted boiling water for about 12 minutes, or according to the packet instructions.
3. While the pasta is cooking, put the soaked cashews, almond milk, oregano, smoked paprika, half the olive oil, 1 tablespoon water and a sprinkling of sea salt and black pepper in a food processor and blend until smooth and creamy.
4. In a large, non-stick frying pan, gently fry the mushrooms in the remaining olive oil for 5–6 minutes until softened. Add the garlic and fry for 2 minutes.
5. Drain the pasta and return it to its pan, along with the mushrooms and garlic and the creamy sauce. Mix well. If the mixture seems a little dry, add a splash of kettle water and give it all a good toss.
6. Serve with the vegan Parmesan and parsley (if using).

Carbs 53.4g

Calories 587

Fat 29g

Protein 30.1g

Cauliflower Pizza

I think I've made the best recipe for the crispiest vegan cauliflower pizza base ever. I have suggested some toppings (which are included in the calories), but you can easily switch these up to include some vegan meat, chargrilled vegetables or different vegan cheeses – the world is your (vegan) oyster!

MAKES 1 PIZZA

FOR THE BASE
1 cauliflower
10g whole chia seeds
8 fresh basil leaves, finely chopped
1 tbsp cornflour
15g vegan Parmesan, grated
1 tsp sea salt
Freshly ground black pepper

SUGGESTED TOPPINGS
1 tbsp vegan red pesto
30g roasted peppers (from a jar)
50g vegan mozzarella, sliced
Dried chilli flakes (optional)
Fresh basil leaves

1. Preheat the oven to 190°C/375°F/Gas 5. Line a baking sheet with non-stick baking paper.
2. Grab the cauliflower and grate the tops of the florets into a bowl, discarding the tougher stems. Bring a saucepan of water to the boil, add the grated cauliflower and cook for 5 minutes until just tender. Line a sieve with a tea towel and pour the contents of the pan through it. Leave to cool.
3. Place the chia seeds in a small spice blender and blitz until ground. Mix with 60ml water and set aside for 5 minutes to make a chia 'egg'.
4. Twist the tea towel with the cauliflower in it to squeeze out any excess water. Take care as the water may still be hot. Try to get as much excess water out as possible as this is the trick for getting a crispy base.
5. In a large bowl, use your hands to mix together the cauliflower rice, chia 'egg', basil, cornflour, vegan Parmesan and some sea salt and black pepper. If the mixture isn't coming together, add a dash of water.
6. Tip the mixture on to the lined baking sheet and press into a circular shape, just over 1cm thick. Bake in the oven for 35–40 minutes until crisp and golden.
7. Remove the pizza base from the oven and spread the red pesto over it. Slice the peppers and add them to the base, along with the vegan cheese. Cook the pizza for a further 10–15 minutes, or until the toppings are hot. Sprinkle with basil leaves and chilli flakes (if using).

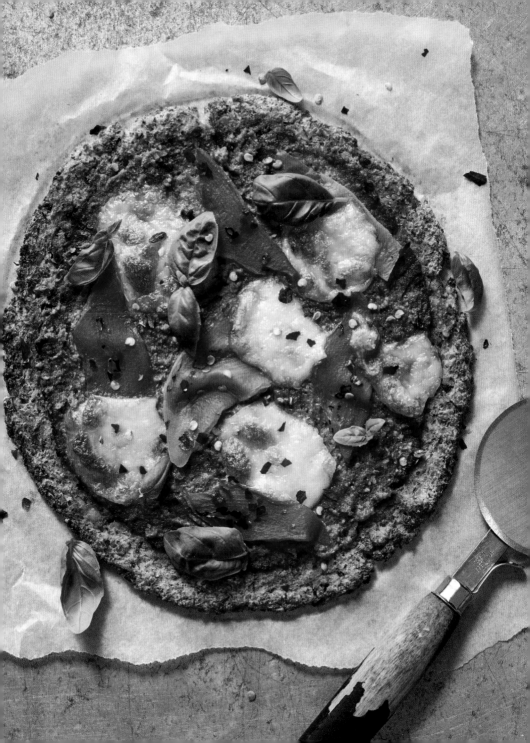

Carbs 40g

Calories 336

Fat 9.9g

Protein 19.8g

Crispy Tofu Nuggets

These are a vegan version of crispy chicken nuggets and can be eaten as a snack, a starter or served with salad and potatoes for a more substantial meal.

SERVES 4

350g extra-firm tofu
120ml plant-based milk
1½ tbsp cornflour
180g breadcrumbs
2 tsp smoked paprika
2 tsp garlic powder
Pinch of sea salt
Pinch of freshly ground
    black pepper
70g plain flour
Favourite dipping sauce,
    to serve

1. Preheat the oven to 200°C/400°F/Gas 6.
2. Slice the block of tofu into three large rectangles and lay on a sheet of kitchen paper with a second piece on top. Weigh this down, using a heavy book or pot and allow the excess water to slowly drain out. This can be done for anything from an hour to overnight, if left in the fridge.
3. Once the excess water has been removed, break the tofu slices into chunks, similar in size to nuggets, weighing roughly 20g each.
4. In a bowl, mix together the plant-based milk and cornflour until smooth. In a separate bowl, mix the breadcrumbs, smoked paprika, garlic powder, sea salt and pepper.
5. Take each chunk of tofu, dredge in the flour and tap against the side of the bowl to remove any excess. Next, drop them into the milk mixture, again allowing the excess to drip off. Finally, dip the tofu into the breadcrumb mixture, pressing them into the bowl until evenly coated.
6. Lay each nugget on a wire rack on a baking tray. Cook in the oven for 15–20 minutes until golden and crisp. Serve hot with your favourite dipping sauce.

Carbs 41.6g

Calories 462

Fat 16.4g

Protein 9.1g

Vegan Buffalo Cauliflower Tacos

These soft tacos are packed full of spicy buffalo sauce, crispy cauliflower, avocado and delicious salad. They are a winner, even for the most seasoned meat eater.

SERVES 2
2 tbsp plain flour
90ml plant-based milk
1 tsp garlic powder
1 tsp paprika
½ cauliflower head, broken into florets
1 tbsp olive oil (or coconut oil)
1 tbsp maple syrup
3 tbsp buffalo hot sauce
1 corn-on-the-cob (around 100g)
4 mini white tortilla wraps
Handful of lettuce, torn into pieces
½ avocado, sliced
½ red onion, finely sliced
Small handful of fresh coriander leaves, torn
1 tbsp vegan yoghurt (e.g. soya)
Sea salt
Freshly ground black pepper

1. Preheat the oven to 230°C/450°F/Gas 8. Line a baking tray with non-stick baking paper.
2. In a large bowl, mix together the plain flour, plant-based milk, garlic powder, paprika and some sea salt and black pepper.
3. Add the cauliflower florets to the bowl and mix to combine. Make sure every piece of the cauliflower is coated in the batter.
4. Place the cauliflower on the lined tray. Try to make sure that the florets aren't touching each other, so that they crisp nicely. Bake for 20 minutes, turning each floret over halfway through cooking.
5. In a jug or small bowl, mix together the olive (or coconut) oil, maple syrup and buffalo hot sauce. Stir until well combined.
6. Remove the cauliflower florets from the oven and brush the hot sauce mixture over each one until well coated. Bake for a further 20 minutes.
7. Stand the corn cob vertically on a chopping board and, with a sharp knife, slice down the sides so that the sweetcorn falls off. Heat a non-stick frying pan on a high heat without any oil and fry the corn until nicely charred, stirring occasionally. Set aside.
8. Assemble the tacos by layering some lettuce inside each wrap, then top with avocado and red onion, finishing with the buffalo cauliflower and some fresh coriander. Drizzle over some vegan yoghurt and serve.

Carbs 49.1g

Calories 530

Fat 24g

Protein 30.1g

Vegan Meatball Pasta

You would be forgiven for thinking that these meatballs aren't vegan – they taste just like the real thing!

SERVES 4

2 tsp olive oil
1 onion, finely chopped
2 garlic cloves, finely chopped
1 tsp dried oregano
1 tbsp ground flaxseed
500g vegan sausages (from the chilled aisle)
1 tbsp vegan Parmesan, grated
Handful of fresh basil
65g breadcrumbs
2 heaped tsp tomato purée
260g spaghetti
Sea salt
Freshly ground black pepper
Sea salt
Freshly ground black pepper
Large handful of rocket leaves, to serve

1. Preheat the oven to 200°C/400°F/Gas 6. Line a baking tray with non-stick baking paper.
2. Heat the olive oil in a frying pan over a medium heat and add the onion and garlic. Gently fry for about 5–6 minutes until softened and beginning to colour. Add the oregano and cook for a further minute.
3. Mix the flaxseed with 2 tablespoons water in a small bowl to make a flaxseed 'egg' and set aside.
4. Remove the skins from the sausages (if skin-on vegan sausages) and break the filling into chunks. Tip the sausage meat into a food processor, along with the onion and garlic mixture, Parmesan and basil. Blitz until nearly smooth.
5. Transfer to a bowl, along with the flaxseed 'egg', the breadcrumbs, tomato purée and salt and pepper and mix together.
6. Divide the mixture into roughly sixteen balls and place them on the lined baking tray. Bake on the middle shelf of the oven for 15–20 minutes until they are piping hot in the middle.
7. While the meatballs are cooking, prepare the sauce. Heat a frying pan with the olive oil over a low heat. Add the garlic and gently fry for 1–2 minutes. Add the chilli flakes and stir for another minute.

FOR THE SAUCE
1 tsp olive oil
1 garlic clove, finely sliced
Pinch of dried chilli flakes
2 × 400g tins chopped
   tomatoes
1 tsp maple syrup

8. Add the tomatoes and maple syrup to the pan and crush with a wooden spoon. Turn the heat up to medium–high and simmer gently to reduce. Season with sea salt and black pepper to taste.
9. Bring a saucepan of salted water to the boil and add the spaghetti. Cook according to the packet instructions.
10. Once cooked, drain and stir through the sauce. Serve with the baked meatballs on top of the spaghetti and scatter over the rocket leaves to finish.

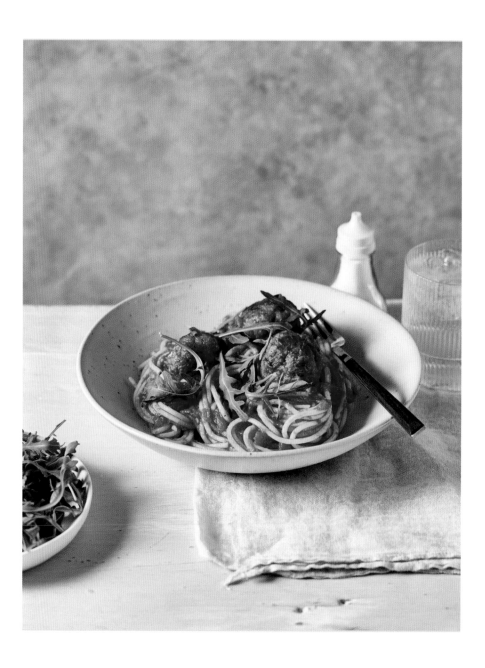

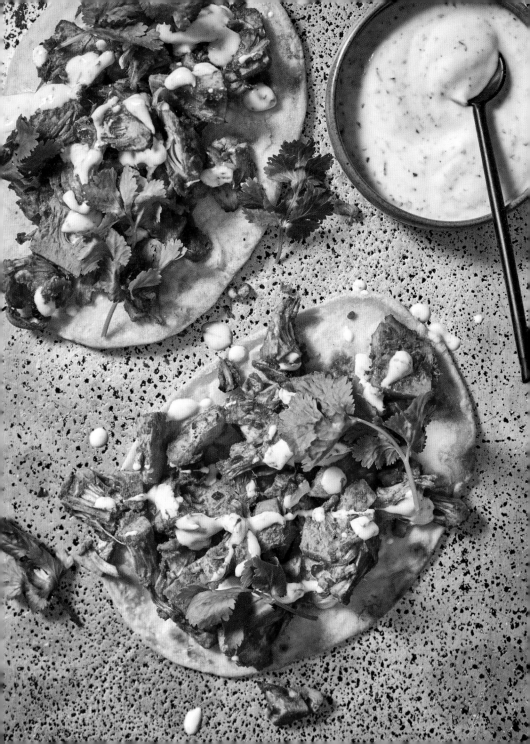

Carbs 53.2g

Calories 361

Fat 10.9g

Protein 9.4g

Vegan Jackfruit Kebabs with Flatbreads

These are unbelievably delicious. The meaty jackfruit makes for a perfect low-calorie and vegan kebab alternative. I've paired them with a really quick and simple garlic and mint sauce (to cool the heat of the kebabs), as well as giving you a quick flatbread recipe, which works really well with the other flavours here.

MAKES 2

FOR THE JACKFRUIT KEBABS
1 × 410g tin jackfruit (200g drained weight)
1 tsp smoked paprika
1 tsp ground cumin
1 tsp ground coriander
½ tsp dried chilli flakes
2 tsp olive oil
2 tsp tomato purée
1 tsp garlic purée (or 2 garlic cloves, minced)
1 tsp maple syrup
2 tsp low-sodium soy sauce

1. To make the kebabs, drain and rinse the jackfruit, remove any visible seeds and cut off the hard, pointy ends. Slice the chunks lengthways and place in a mixing bowl.
2. Add the smoked paprika, ground cumin and coriander and chilli flakes and mix together.
3. Heat a frying pan over a medium heat and add the olive oil. Add the seasoned jackfruit to the pan and sauté for 3–4 minutes. Mix in the tomato and garlic purées, maple syrup and soy sauce and stir to combine. Add 25ml water and mix again, scraping the base of the pan.
4. Reduce the heat and gently simmer for 10 minutes. Squash the jackfruit with the back of a spoon until you have flaky, chunky pieces. Once the liquid has reduced, take off the heat, tip on to a baking tray lined with non-stick baking paper and spread the pieces out evenly.
5. To finish cooking, grill the jackfruit for 10 minutes under a medium heat until the edges are crispy and golden.

FOR THE FLATBREADS
100g plain flour, plus extra
   for kneading and rolling
½ tsp sea salt
50ml warm water
½ tbsp olive oil
Low-calorie cooking spray

**FOR THE GARLIC AND
MINT SAUCE**
200g vegan yoghurt (soya
   or coconut)
½ tbsp mint sauce
1 tsp garlic purée

6. Next, make the flatbreads. Combine the flour and salt in a mixing bowl and slowly add the water, little by little, mixing together.

7. Add the olive oil and knead the dough until you have a smooth, soft consistency. If it is too dry, add a splash more water and knead again. Turn the dough out on to a lightly floured surface and knead for 5 minutes, then pop it into a clean bowl and cover with cling film or a tea towel and leave for 10–30 minutes, or until you are ready to cook the flatbreads.

8. When you are ready, divide the dough into two balls. Sprinkle a little flour on to a clean surface and flatten the balls out into circles using a rolling pin. Add a little more flour to the top (to ensure they don't stick) and flip over. Roll them out to roughly the thickness of a pound coin.

9. Heat a large frying pan over a medium–high heat. Spray a few times with low-calorie spray and wipe around the pan with a piece of kitchen paper. Cook each flatbread for 2–3 minutes on each side. You should see them puff up slightly and char in patches.

10. To make the garlic and mint sauce, simply mix the yoghurt, mint sauce and garlic purée in a small bowl until well combined.

11. Top the flatbreads with the jackfruit kebab and drizzle with garlic and mint sauce to serve.

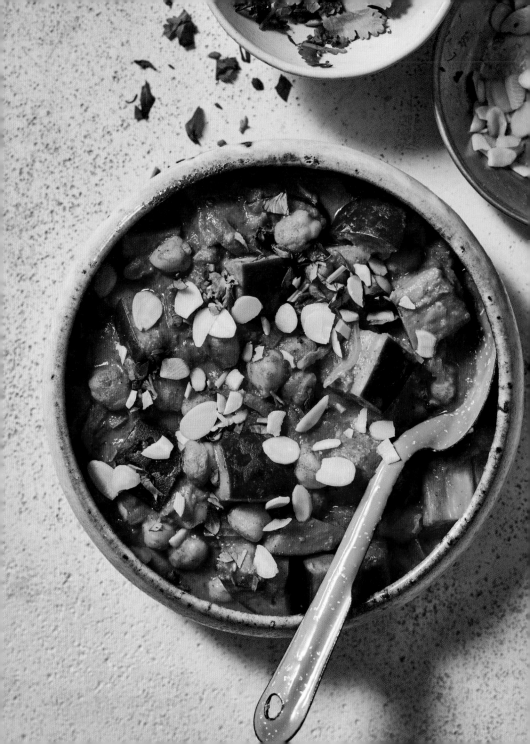

Carbs 19.2g

Calories 294

Fat 15.2g

Protein 7.9g

Aubergine and Chickpea Curry

Aubergines are a great way to get more fibre into your diet. They are filling, yet low-fat and they help to reduce cholesterol, too. Along with the delicious spices, they make the perfect simple vegan curry.

SERVES 4

1 tbsp olive oil
2 red onions, finely sliced
3 garlic cloves, finely chopped
Thumb-sized piece of fresh ginger, grated
½ tsp dried chilli flakes
2 tsp ground cumin
2 tsp ground coriander
2 tsp garam masala
1 tsp ground turmeric
2 tsp medium curry powder
1 × 400g tin chopped tomatoes
2 aubergines, cut into large cubes
1 × 400g tin chickpeas, drained and rinsed
1 × 400g tin light coconut milk
1 tbsp flaked almonds
½ bunch fresh coriander leaves
Sea salt
Freshly ground black pepper

1. Heat the olive oil in a large, non-stick saucepan over a medium heat and fry the onions until cooked down and softened.
2. Add the garlic and ginger and fry for a further minute before adding all the spices and a splash of water. Stir for a minute until fragrant, then add the tomatoes.
3. Lower the heat to reduce the liquid a little (for about 5 minutes) before adding the aubergines and chickpeas. Stir, then cover with a lid and simmer for about 10 minutes until the aubergine is soft. If the mixture is looking a little thick, add a splash of water to stop it catching on the base of the pan.
4. Remove the lid and pour in the coconut milk and stir. Simmer for 5 minutes until the curry is thick. Season with a little sea salt and black pepper.
5. Serve, garnished with the almonds and coriander.

Carbs 30.8g	
Calories 420	
Fat 12.8g	
Protein 27.2g	

Veggie Moussaka

Packed full of healthy vegetables and finished with a thick layer of cheesy white sauce, this is the ultimate comfort food and a true Greek experience.

SERVES 6

1 tbsp olive oil
2 onions, finely chopped
2 garlic cloves, finely chopped
2 tsp ground cinnamon
1 tsp allspice
400g vegetarian 'mince'
2 × 400g tins chopped tomatoes
1 × 400g tin chickpeas, drained and rinsed
1 tbsp tomato purée
1 vegetable stock cube
1 tsp dried oregano
650g potatoes, peeled and cut into slices 1cm thick
400ml skimmed milk
2 tbsp cornflour
½ tsp grated nutmeg
200g reduced-fat soft cheese
2 aubergines, thinly sliced
100g reduced-fat feta cheese
30g Parmesan, grated
Sea salt
Freshly ground black pepper

1. Preheat the oven to 190°C/375°F/Gas 5.
2. Place the oil in a large frying pan, then add the onions and fry over a medium heat for about 5–8 minutes until softened.
3. Add the garlic to the pan, along with the cinnamon and allspice. Cook for another minute, stirring often, until fragrant, then add the 'mince' and reduce the heat a little. Season with salt and pepper and cook for another minute or so, stirring to prevent the mince from catching.
4. Add the chopped tomatoes, chickpeas and tomato purée, then half-fill a tin with water and add that, along with the stock cube (crumbled) and oregano. Simmer for 10–15 minutes until the sauce has thickened.
5. Add the potatoes to a large saucepan of boiling water and cook for 3 minutes until nearly soft, but not falling apart. Drain and set aside.
6. To make the white sauce topping, add a splash of the milk (about 1 tablespoon) to the cornflour and mix together. In a small saucepan, bring the rest of the milk to a simmer over a medium heat before seasoning with the nutmeg and pouring in the cornflour mixture. Add the soft cheese and whisk thoroughly until thick and smooth.
7. To assemble the moussaka, pour one half of the 'mince' sauce into an ovenproof dish. Layer with half the aubergine slices and potatoes and crumble over half the feta. Top with the rest of the 'mince' and a second layer of aubergine, potato and feta. Finish with a layer of white sauce and top with the grated Parmesan. Bake for 30–40 minutes until bubbling and golden.

Carbs 67.9g

Calories 450

Fat 5.3g

Protein 21.1g

Perfect Vegan Bean Burger

It's difficult to find a good-quality vegan burger that actually tastes nice, but this one changes all that. High in protein and low in fat, here's a burger that will make you want to go back for more.

SERVES 2

½ tbsp ground flaxseed (a vegan alternative to eggs, for binding the mixture)
1 × 400g tin mixed beans, drained and rinsed
Small handful of coriander, stalks and leaves chopped
1 tub fresh salsa
1 garlic clove, finely grated
1 tsp olive oil
½ lime
½ tsp dried chilli flakes
Pinch of sea salt
70g breadcrumbs
2 wholemeal vegan burger buns
1 Little Gem lettuce, sliced

1. Preheat the oven to 200°C/400°F/Gas 6. Line a baking tray with non-stick baking paper.
2. To make the flax 'egg', mix the ground flaxseed with 1¼ tablespoons water in a small bowl.
3. In a food processor, blitz half the beans, the flax 'egg', coriander, a small tablespoonful of the salsa, the garlic and olive oil until nearly smooth.
4. In a bowl, lightly break up the remaining beans with a fork, then add the blitzed bean mixture, a squeeze of lime juice, the chilli flakes and salt. Mix together with your hands, then add the breadcrumbs, little by little, until the mixture comes together and has a good consistency for shaping. Divide the mixture into two balls and shape into patties.
5. Transfer to the lined baking tray and cook in the oven for 20 minutes, turning halfway through.
6. Assemble your burgers with the burger buns, a little of the salsa and lettuce leaves.

BUDGET MEALS

Quick Tuna Burgers

The ultimate cupboard food – you only need some tinned ingredients (and a few fresh) and you're ready to go. These are absolutely divine and the kids will love them!

SERVES 4
70g breadcrumbs
2 × 145g tins tuna, drained
3 spring onions, finely chopped
1 × 198g tin sweetcorn, drained
2 free-range eggs, beaten
1 tbsp olive oil
Sea salt
Freshly ground black pepper

FOR THE RED ONION PICKLE
1 red onion, finely sliced
1 tsp maple syrup
3 tbsp red wine vinegar (or white wine vinegar)
1 tsp sea salt
Boiling water

TO SERVE
4 burger buns
Tomato ketchup (or sauce of your choice)
1 Little Gem lettuce, bottom sliced off
1 large tomato, sliced
½ cucumber, sliced

1. Firstly, get on with the pickle. In a small bowl, mix together the onion, maple syrup, vinegar and sea salt and pour over enough boiling water to cover. Stir with a fork and set aside to pickle while you make the tuna burgers.
2. Put the breadcrumbs, tuna, half the spring onions and half the sweetcorn in a large bowl.
3. In a food processor, blitz the remaining sweetcorn and spring onions until finely chopped. Add to the bowl. Season well with sea salt and black pepper and mix everything well with your hands.
4. Slowly add the beaten eggs, bit by bit, until the mixture forms one large ball. Divide the mixture into four burger patties.
5. Heat the oil in a frying pan and fry the burgers for 2–3 minutes on each side until golden brown and beginning to crisp.
6. To assemble the burgers, simply toast the buns and then add your favourite sauce. Top with the lettuce, a tomato slice, then the tuna burger and the cucumber.
7. Grab some red onion pickle, shaking off any excess moisture and add to the burger to finish.

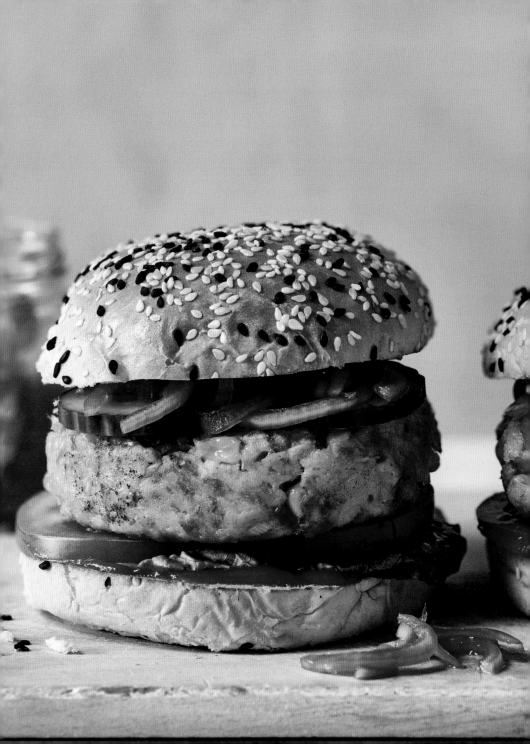

Carbs 38g

Calories 370

Fat 25.3g

Protein 37.2g

Beef Hot Pot

This dish just gives me all the feels: it is comforting and warming – and the addition of crispy potatoes on top makes it the best hot-pot recipe around.

SERVES 4
1 tbsp olive oil
500g extra-lean beef
　mince
1 onion, finely diced
1 large carrot, peeled and
　finely diced
3 garlic cloves, finely
　sliced
1 tsp chopped fresh
　rosemary leaves
1 bay leaf
1 tbsp tomato purée
½ tbsp balsamic vinegar
1 tsp Worcestershire
　sauce
1 tsp mint sauce
1 tsp honey
450ml beef or chicken
　stock
100g frozen peas
900g potatoes, peeled
　and sliced to around
　1.5cm thickness
Low-calorie cooking spray
Sea salt
Freshly ground black
　pepper

1. Preheat the oven to 200°C/400°F/Gas 6.
2. In a large, non-stick frying pan, heat the olive oil over a medium–high heat and fry the mince, onion and carrot for 10–15 minutes until the mince is browned and the vegetables are beginning to tenderise. Stir in the garlic and fry for a further 2 minutes.
3. Stir in the rosemary, bay leaf, tomato purée, balsamic vinegar, Worcestershire sauce, mint sauce and honey.
4. Pour in the stock and bring to the boil. Once boiling, reduce the heat to low and simmer for 15 minutes until thickened. Season with salt and pepper to taste.
5. Stir in the frozen peas, then transfer to an ovenproof casserole dish. Lay the potato slices on the top, overlapping them slightly, until you have covered the entire top of the mixture.
6. Spray the top of the potatoes with cooking spray and season again with salt. Bake in the oven for about 40–50 minutes until the potatoes are tender and golden and the vegetables are cooked.

Carbs 49.1g

Calories 530

Fat 24g

Protein 30.1g

Creamy Chicken Jacket Potato

This meal is cheap, but it's also totally delicious. Creamy chicken sauce spooned over a piping hot jacket potato is anyone's idea of comfort food.

MAKES 2
2 large baking potatoes
1 boneless, skinless chicken breast
100g reduced-fat garlic and herb soft cheese
1 tbsp fat-free yoghurt
1 tbsp reduced-fat mayonnaise
2 spring onions, finely sliced
½ small red onion, finely chopped
100g sweetcorn
½ tsp Dijon mustard
½ tsp cayenne pepper
Sea salt
Freshly ground black pepper

1. Preheat the oven to 200°C/400°F/Gas 6.
2. Place the potatoes on a baking tray, sprinkle with a little salt and pepper and bake in the oven for 1 hour.
3. While the potatoes are baking, wrap the chicken breast in foil, and after the potatoes have been cooking for 20 minutes, transfer the chicken breast parcel to the oven – they should finish cooking at the same time.
4. Once the chicken is cooked through (when it is no longer pink and the juices run clear), remove from the oven and then shred it into chunky pieces in a bowl using two forks.
5. In a separate bowl, mix together the soft cheese, yoghurt, mayonnaise, spring onions, red onion, sweetcorn and mustard. Add the shredded chicken to the dressing and stir to combine.
6. Cut a slit in the top of each of the baked potatoes and pull apart. Scoop out and discard a little flesh from the potatoes and fill them with the chicken mixture.
7. Sprinkle over the cayenne pepper and enjoy!

Sweet Potato Curry with Easy Naans

Sweet potatoes are nutritional powerhouses – full of fibre, vitamins and minerals, they promote gut health, support healthy vision and enhance brain function. Instead of rice, this curry is paired with some delicious, quick homemade naans. Make them vegan by simply using a yoghurt alternative.

SERVES 6

2 large sweet potatoes, peeled and cut into 2cm chunks
4 red peppers, deseeded and cut into 2cm chunks
Low-calorie cooking spray
2 tbsp garam masala
2 tbsp ground cumin
1 large onion, sliced
3 garlic cloves, finely chopped
2 × 400g tins chopped tomatoes
150ml vegetable stock
1 tsp honey
4 large handfuls of fresh baby spinach
Sea salt
Freshly ground black pepper

FOR THE NAANS

250g plain flour
250g yoghurt (or vegan alternative)
2 tsp baking powder
½ tsp sea salt

1. Preheat the oven to 180°C/350°F/Gas 4.
2. Place the sweet potatoes and red peppers on a large baking tray and spray all over with the low-calorie cooking spray. Season with sea salt and black pepper, sprinkle over half the garam masala and half the cumin and bake for 15 minutes.
3. Heat a few more sprays of low-calorie cooking spray in a large, non-stick frying pan over a medium heat and fry the onion for 3–5 minutes until softened and beginning to turn golden.
4. Add the garlic and fry for a further 1–2 minutes until fragrant. Add the remaining garam masala and cumin and stir, cooking for 1 minute.
5. Add the tomatoes and stock and bring to the boil, then reduce the heat to a simmer and cook for 25 minutes.
6. When the sweet potatoes and peppers are cooked, add them to the curry and simmer for a further 10 minutes until the liquid has reduced and the vegetables are tender.
7. For the final 4–5 minutes, spoon in the honey and then add the spinach, allowing it to wilt in the curry.
8. To make the naans, mix all the ingredients in a bowl with your hands. Continue to work the mixture until it comes together as a dough. If it is too sticky, keep adding small amounts of plain flour until it is very easy to handle.
9. Remove the dough from the bowl and split into six portions. Roll each portion out on a floured surface with

a rolling pin to your desired thickness. The thinner you make the dough, the crispier it will become when fried.

10. Fry each naan in a hot dry frying pan until golden and puffed up. This should take a few minutes on each side.

11. Before serving, taste the curry and season with sea salt and black pepper. Serve with the easy naans.

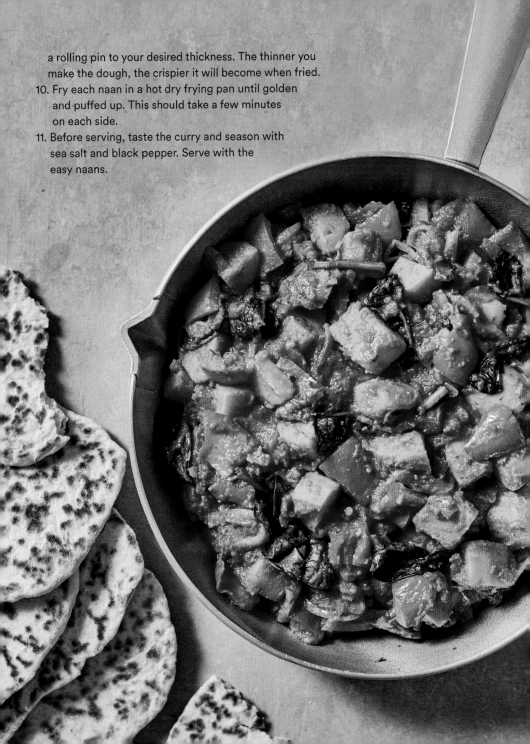

Carbs 23.4g

Calories 220

Fat 4.7g

Protein 22.9g

Grandma's Fish Pie

To make this meal healthier, and also to skip an entire step, I swapped the mash potato topping for thin, crispy potatoes. You'll thank me!

SERVES 6

550g potatoes, peeled and sliced to 5mm thickness
1 large onion, finely chopped
Low-calorie cooking spray
2 garlic cloves, finely chopped
50g plain flour
50g low-fat spread
400ml skimmed milk
Zest of 1 lemon
600g frozen fish pie mix (salmon, cod, haddock, prawns, etc.)
100g frozen peas
150g baby spinach
Sea salt
Freshly ground black pepper

1. Preheat the oven to 190°C/375°F/Gas 5.
2. Boil the sliced potatoes for 2 minutes in salted water, being careful not to break them. Drain and set aside.
3. Place the onion in a large, non-stick saucepan with a few sprays of low-calorie cooking spray over a medium heat and fry for 4–6 minutes until softened. Add the garlic and fry for a further 2 minutes.
4. Sprinkle over the flour and stir through, then add the low-fat spread, cooking for 1–2 minutes. Slowly add the milk, a ladleful at a time, stirring well, until the sauce has thickened. Season with sea salt and freshly ground black pepper, then grate in some lemon zest.
5. Turn the heat off and add the fish-pie mix, stirring well. Add the frozen peas and baby spinach and stir again.
6. Pour the mixture into an ovenproof dish and lay the sliced potatoes on top. Spray with more cooking spray.
7. Bake for 30–40 minutes until the fish is cooked and the potatoes are crisp and golden. Serve with your favourite green vegetables.

Carbs 59.6g

Calories 584

Fat 14g

Protein 50.8g

Chicken Kiev with Truffle and Parmesan Fries

There is no more perfect combination than crisp, juicy chicken filled with a buttery, garlic sauce. I've even teamed these Kievs with some crispy truffle fries.

SERVES 2

1 tbsp reduced-fat soft cheese

1 tbsp low-fat spread

2 garlic cloves, finely grated

1 tbsp finely chopped parsley

2 boneless, skinless chicken breasts

2 tbsp plain flour

1 free-range egg, beaten

40g breadcrumbs

2 potatoes, sliced into 5mm matchsticks

Low-calorie cooking spray

1 tsp truffle oil

30g Parmesan, grated

Salad leaves, to serve

Sea salt

Freshly ground black pepper

1. Preheat the oven to 200°C/400°F/Gas 6.
2. In a small bowl, mix together the soft cheese, low-fat spread, garlic and parsley.
3. Slice a pocket into the thick side of each chicken breast and push the garlic filling into it, taking care not to put a hole straight through the chicken.
4. In three different bowls, set out the flour (seasoned with salt and pepper), beaten egg and breadcrumbs. Dip the chicken breasts into the flour, then the egg. Shake off the excess and then sprinkle with a coating of breadcrumbs. Chill in the fridge for 15 minutes while you get on with your fries.
5. Place the potato matchsticks in a pan of boiling water and boil for 3 minutes. Remove, drain and rinse in cold water. Pat dry.
6. Spray a large baking tray about ten times with cooking spray and add the fries in a single layer, ensuring they are not touching each other. Add another five sprays of cooking spray and sprinkle with salt and black pepper.
7. Bake the fries in the oven for 40 minutes, flipping halfway through.
8. At the same time, transfer the Kievs to the oven and bake for 35–40 minutes until cooked through (when the chicken is no longer pink and the juices run clear).
9. When the fries are cooked, remove from the oven and stir through the truffle oil and top with the grated Parmesan. Serve with the kievs and a side salad.

Carbs 49.1g

Calories 356

Fat 8.2g

Protein 21.5g

Garlic Prawn Stir-fry

What better dish to celebrate the great king prawn than a delicious, quick stir-fry? Prawns are a great source of low-fat protein. They also contain a good amount of selenium, which we need to maintain cell health, and they're full of zinc, which is crucial for a healthy immune system.

SERVES 2

150g wholewheat noodles (or regular)

1 tbsp olive oil

1 red onion, finely chopped

1 red pepper, deseeded and sliced

5 garlic cloves, finely chopped

Thumb-sized piece of fresh ginger, peeled and finely sliced into matchsticks

1 red chilli, deseeded and finely sliced

1 carrot, sliced into matchsticks

100g Tenderstem broccoli tips

8 sugar snap peas

165 raw king prawns (try to get jumbo size)

1 tbsp low-sodium soy sauce

1 tbsp honey

Juice of ½ lime

1 tsp Chinese five-spice

½ bunch fresh coriander leaves

1. Cook the noodles in a pan of boiling water, according to the packet instructions, then drain and set aside. If you are using fresh noodles, skip this step for now.
2. In a large, non-stick frying pan (or wok), heat the olive oil over a high heat. Once hot, add the onion and red pepper to the pan and cook, stirring constantly, for 1 minute.
3. Add the garlic, ginger and chilli and fry for 1 minute. Add the carrot, broccoli and sugar snaps to the pan and stir-fry for a further 2 minutes until the colours of the vegetables intensify.
4. Add the prawns and, as soon as they turn pink, pour in the soy sauce, honey, lime juice and five-spice. Add a splash of water and reduce the heat slightly.
5. Add the noodles and give everything a good mix. If you are using fresh noodles, cook them in the stir-fry, according to the packet instructions.
6. Serve with lots of scattered coriander leaves.

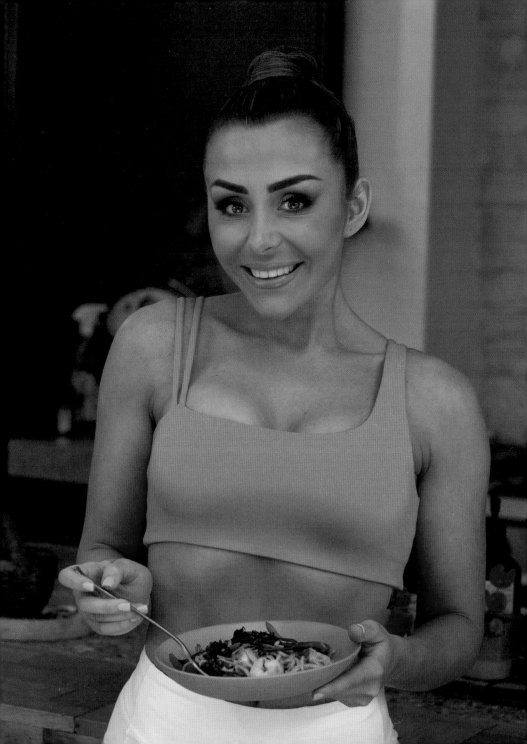

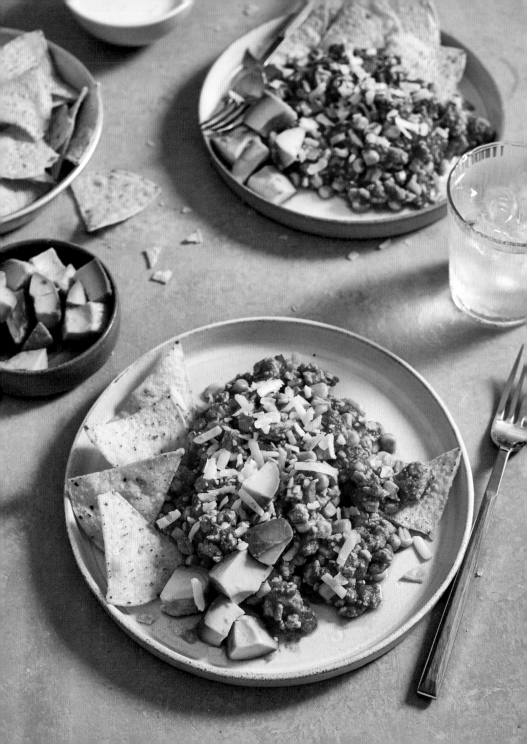

Carbs 29.2g

Calories 385

Fat 13.9g

Protein 37.4g

Turkey Chili

This turkey chili is smoky and meaty with the perfect kick, and it's an ideal way to use up store-cupboard items. I use turkey mince here for an extra dose of protein, but you could easily substitute beef mince – just make sure you use the lean variety.

SERVES 4

1 tbsp olive oil
500g 2%-fat turkey mince
1 large onion, finely diced
1 red pepper, deseeded
 and finely diced
4 garlic cloves, finely
 chopped
1 tsp smoked paprika
½ tsp cayenne pepper
2 tsp ground cumin
1 tsp hot chilli powder
1 tsp ground coriander
1 tsp dried oregano
1 cinnamon stick, bashed
1 tbsp tomato ketchup
1 tbsp BBQ sauce
1 × 340g tin sweetcorn,
 drained
1 × 400g tin chopped
 tomatoes
1 chicken stock cube
300ml boiling water
Sea salt
Freshly ground black
 pepper

TO SERVE

20 tortilla chips
4 tbsp fat-free yoghurt
½ avocado, sliced into
 chunks
Grated cheese of your
 choice

1. In a large, non-stick frying pan, heat the oil over a medium–high heat and fry the turkey mince for about 10 minutes until browned all over and beginning to crackle.
2. Remove the mince from the pan and add the onion and red pepper. Fry for 4–5 minutes until softened and beginning to turn golden. Add the garlic and fry for a further 2 minutes.
3. Add the smoked paprika, cayenne pepper, cumin, chilli powder, ground coriander and oregano. Stir well until combined. Add the cinnamon stick.
4. Add the ketchup, BBQ sauce, sweetcorn, chopped tomatoes, stock cube and water. Stir well and season with sea salt and black pepper.
5. Return the turkey mince to the pan and bring to a vigorous simmer, then reduce the heat and leave to simmer gently for 40 minutes until reduced and thickened.
6. Serve with the tortilla chips, yoghurt, avocado and cheese (if using).

Carbs 56.1g

Calories 396

Fat 5.6g

Protein 20.6g

Lentil Bolognese

Full of soluble fibre, lentils are a nutritional powerhouse which help to reduce cholesterol, aid your digestive system and provide a good source of plant protein. This dish tastes just like a meat alternative and can be easily meal-prepped and then frozen for later.

SERVES 4

1 tbsp olive oil
1 carrot, finely diced
1 onion, finely diced
1 celery stick, finely diced
3 garlic cloves, finely
  chopped
1 tsp dried oregano
250g dried red lentils
1 tsp maple syrup
1 tbsp tomato purée
1 × 400g tin chopped
  tomatoes
1 bay leaf
1 vegetable stock cube
800ml boiling water
300g dried spaghetti
Sea salt
Freshly ground black
  pepper
Side salad, to serve

1. Place the olive oil in a large saucepan over a medium heat. Add the carrot, onion and celery and fry for about 10 minutes until slightly softened.

2. Add the garlic and stir, frying for a further 2 minutes. Sprinkle over the dried oregano and fry for another 2 minutes.

3. Pour in the lentils, maple syrup, tomato purée, chopped tomatoes, bay leaf, stock cube and boiling water. Season with sea salt and black pepper.

4. Stir well, then turn the heat down to medium–low and leave to simmer for 30–35 minutes, ensuring that the lentils do not stick at the bottom of the pan. If they begin to stick, the heat is too high. Cook until the lentils are tender and the sauce has thickened.

5. While the sauce is simmering, cook the pasta in salted boiling water for 12 minutes (or according to the packet instructions).

6. To serve, mix the sauce through the spaghetti and serve with a side salad.

Carbs 68g	
Calories 448	
Fat 15.1g	
Protein 24.5g	

Roasted Tomato and Mozzarella Pasta

Sweet tomatoes and gooey garlic tossed through fibre-rich wholewheat spaghetti . . . There is a slight kick from the chilli flakes, but the cool, creamy mozzarella takes the heat down to make a delicious, balanced summer dish that can be eaten all year round. I really recommend using nice, ripe tomatoes for this as the taste will be so much better.

SERVES 4

3 vine tomatoes, halved
3 garlic cloves, skin on
1 red onion, cut into wedges
Low-calorie cooking spray
150g wholewheat spaghetti
½ tsp dried chilli flakes
10 black olives
120g reduced-fat mozzarella
½ bunch fresh basil leaves
Sea salt
Freshly ground black pepper

1. Preheat the oven to 190°C/375°F/Gas 5.
2. Place the tomatoes, garlic and red onion in a small baking tray and spray liberally with the low-calorie cooking spray. Season well with salt and black pepper and bake for 35–40 minutes until soft.
3. Meanwhile, cook the spaghetti in boiling salted water for 12–15 minutes, or according to the packet instructions. Drain well.
4. Return the pasta to the pan and stir through the roasted tomatoes and the red onion, chilli flakes and black olives. The garlic cloves can be squeezed out of their skins and mixed through, too (optional).
5. Serve in large bowls, topped with torn mozzarella and basil leaves.

TOP TIP: don't keep your tomatoes in the fridge. Leave them on a sunny windowsill and the flavour will develop naturally.

SWEET TREATS

Apple Pie Tarts

With delicious puff pastry, sweet apple filling and warming spice, these apple-pie tarts are just as tasty as their higher-calorie counterparts.

MAKES 4

2 red apples, peeled and cut into 1cm chunks
1 tsp ground cinnamon, plus extra to garnish
4 tsp apple sauce
160g light puff pastry, cut into 4 rectangles

1. Preheat the oven to 170°C/325°F/Gas 3. Line a baking tray with non-stick baking paper.
2. Pour 50ml water into a small saucepan and add the apples. Simmer over a low–medium heat until the apples are soft and the liquid has reduced significantly.
3. Add the cinnamon and apple sauce and stir. Take off the heat and set aside.
4. Score a line down each side of the puff-pastry rectangles, about 1cm from the edge, to form a scored rectangle within each one.
5. Add a dollop of the cooked apple in the centre of the puff-pastry sheets, spreading up to the scored lines.
6. Once all the apple-pie tarts have been assembled, place them on the lined baking tray and bake in the oven for 25 minutes until the pastry is golden and puffed up. Sprinkle over a little cinnamon to serve.

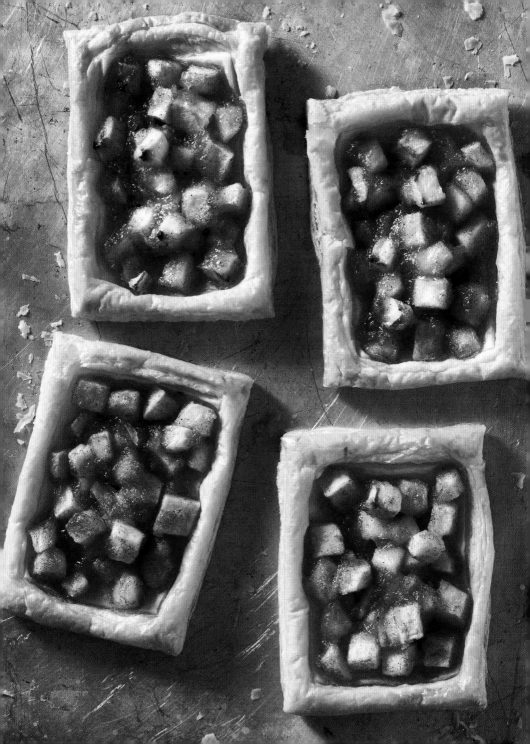

Protein Chocolate Crêpes

These crêpes are so versatile and both kids and adults love them. They can be eaten for breakfast, post work-out or even on Pancake Day. At nearly 13g protein per pancake, they are a much healthier option.

MAKES 4

25g vanilla protein powder
30g plain flour
2 free-range eggs, beaten
20ml semi-skimmed milk
Low-calorie cooking spray
4 tbsp protein chocolate
    spread

1. Sift the protein powder and flour into a large bowl. Add the eggs and milk to the bowl and whisk until well combined.
2. Heat a non-stick frying pan over a medium–high heat, then spray around 5–7 times with cooking spray. Once hot, add a quarter of the batter to the pan, tilting to spread the mixture evenly across the base.
3. Once bubbles begin to form across the surface of the batter, flip the crêpe over and add a tablespoon of the chocolate spread.
4. After 1 minute, roll the crêpe up and repeat the process with the remaining batter.

Carbs 9.2g

Calories 81

Fat 4g

Protein 1.5g

Chocolate and Cinnamon Pastries

These pastries will take your breakfast spread to the next level. Making your own can be difficult, but I've made it super simple and you won't regret giving it a go.

MAKES 16

320g packet light puff pastry
1 heaped tbsp ground cinnamon
1 tsp granulated sweetener
40g chocolate chips
2 tbsp semi-skimmed milk

1. Preheat the oven to 190°C/375°F/Gas 5. Line a baking tray with non-stick baking paper.
2. Roll out the pastry and, using a small brush, splash over a small amount of cold water. Sprinkle over the cinnamon and sweetener as evenly as possible, then sprinkle over the chocolate chips.
3. Take the side closest to you (this should be one of the long sides, not the end) and fold it away from yourself and over the filling. Keep rolling until you have a long pastry tube. Slice into sixteen portions.
4. Place the portions on the lined baking tray, pressing each one down to create a circular shape.
5. Lightly brush a small amount of milk over each one and bake in the oven on a high shelf for 22–25 minutes until golden and puffed up.

Carbs 30g

Calories 180

Fat 5g

Protein 6g

Courtney's Blueberry Scones

A Courtney Black classic, these scones have become a social media sensation. You should definitely try them.

SERVES 6
180g wholemeal flour
1½ tsp baking powder
30g unsalted butter, cut into small pieces
Pinch of sea salt
120g fat-free yoghurt
3 tbsp maple syrup
1 tsp vanilla extract
5 tbsp skimmed milk
80g blueberries
½ tbsp granulated sweetener
Low-fat salted caramel crème fraîche (or butter), to serve

1. Preheat the oven to 200°C/400°F/Gas 6. Line a baking tray with non-stick baking paper.
2. Place the flour, baking powder, butter and salt in a large mixing bowl. Use your fingers to break up, press and mix everything together, as if you are making breadcrumbs.
3. Add the yoghurt, maple syrup, vanilla extract and 3 tablespoons of the milk. Mix together until you have a doughy consistency.
4. Add the blueberries, folding them into the dough with your hands.
5. Tip the dough on to the lined baking tray, mould it into a circular shape and flatten slightly. Brush with the remaining milk and sprinkle over the sweetener to ensure a nice golden finish.
6. Use a knife to score the rounded dough into six sections and bake in the oven for 18–22 minutes, or until golden brown.
7. Once the scone is baked, cut into six portions, then slice through and fill with the crème fraîche.

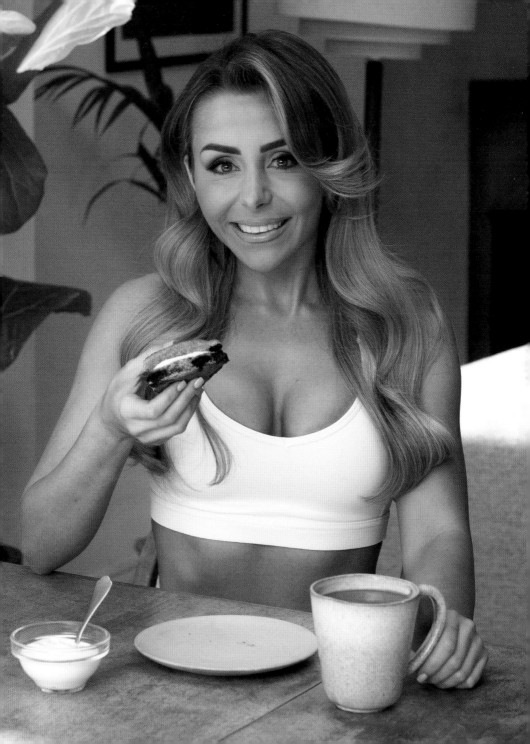

Carbs 29g	
Calories 150	
Fat 1.2g	
Protein 8.2g	

Healthier Jam Doughnuts

These quick and easy doughnuts are so delicious you'd be forgiven for thinking they're high in fat and sugar.

MAKES 4

Low-calorie cooking spray
60g plain flour
1 tsp baking powder
1 tbsp granulated
    sweetener
30g vanilla protein
    powder
White of 1 small free-
    range egg
50g low-fat yoghurt
50ml skimmed milk
2 tsp vanilla extract
25ml maple syrup
4 tsp low-sugar raspberry
    jam
Granulated sweetener,
    for coating

1. Preheat the oven to 200°C/400°F/Gas 6. Lightly spray a muffin tin (a mini hemisphere cake tin works best to give a round doughnut shape when baked, but a small muffin tin will work fine if you don't have one).
2. Sift the flour, baking powder, sweetener and protein powder into a large mixing bowl.
3. Add the egg white, yoghurt, milk, vanilla extract and maple syrup and stir together to make a thick batter.
4. Divide the mixture between four muffin holes, filling nearly to the top, but allowing room for the doughnuts to rise in the oven.
5. Bake for 12–15 minutes, or until cooked through; poke a skewer through one of the doughnuts to check they are done – they will be ready if the skewer comes out clean.
6. Remove from the oven and leave to cool in the tin on a wire rack for at least 10 minutes. While cooling, prepare the filling by thoroughly stirring the jam to create a smooth consistency.
7. Once the doughnuts are cooled, pop them out of the tin. Use a small knife to cut a small whole in the side of each doughnut and spoon or pipe the jam in (a piping bag works best).
8. Arrange on a plate and lightly sift the granulated sweetener over the doughnuts, then turn them over and repeat.

Carbs 25g

Calories 211

Fat 8.3g

Protein 8.8g

Mini Chocolate Lava Cakes

These delicious cakes are dense with a melting middle. Serve them as they are or top with custard or a big scoop of vanilla ice cream.

MAKES 5

30g dark chocolate, chopped
30g milk chocolate, chopped
30g low-fat spread
25g maple syrup
25g sugar-free maple syrup
2 free-range eggs, whisked
3 tbsp (85g) plain flour
25g vanilla protein powder
1 tbsp dark cocoa powder (preferably unsweetened)
Low-calorie cooking spray

1. To melt the chocolate and low-fat spread, place in a medium-sized glass or ceramic heatproof mixing bowl over a pan of simmering water, ensuring that the bottom of the mixing bowl does not touch the water.
2. Slowly stir the chocolate as it begins to melt. Once melted, remove the bowl from the heat and stir in both maple syrups.
3. Whisk the eggs into the chocolate mixture until it forms a smooth batter. Sift in the flour, protein powder and cocoa powder and whisk again.
4. Grease a deep muffin tin with low-calorie cooking spray. Divide the mixture equally between the muffin holes (about 55g per hole) and place the tin in the freezer for about 50–55 minutes (this will ensure gooey centres).
5. Towards the end of the freezing time, preheat the oven to 200°C/400°F/Gas 6.
6. Transfer the tin to the oven and bake for 8–9 minutes. When ready, remove from the oven and leave to cool for 5 minutes (you are looking for a sponge-like cake with a gooey centre).
7. Run a metal spatula or knife around the edges of the muffin holes to release the cakes. Pop them out, turn upside down on to serving plates and serve immediately.

Carbs 27.6g

Calories 162

Fat 2.7g

Protein 6.2g

Blueberry and Yoghurt Loaf Cake

The perfect sponge cake but made so much lighter with the addition of yoghurt. This cake can be eaten as a dessert after dinner or as a slightly naughty breakfast.

SERVES 8
130g low-fat yoghurt
250g self-raising flour
50g maple syrup
4 tbsp granulated sweetener
3 large free-range eggs, beaten
2 tsp vanilla extract
50ml olive oil
25g blueberries
Pinch of sea salt
Low-calorie cooking spray

FOR THE DRIZZLE
2 tsp granulated sweetener
½ tsp vanilla extract

1. Preheat the oven to 180°C/350°F/Gas 4. Spray a loaf tin with the low-calorie cooking spray.
2. In a large bowl, mix together the yoghurt, flour, maple syrup and sweetener until combined.
3. Add the eggs, vanilla, olive oil and a pinch of salt, beating until a smooth batter forms. Fold in the blueberries with a wooden spoon.
4. Pour the batter into the greased loaf tin and bake for 40–55 minutes.
5. While the cake is baking, make the drizzle: place the sweetener in a small cup and stir through the vanilla extract, then add a dash of water to form a syrup.
6. Check the cake is cooked by inserting a wooden skewer into the centre. If it comes out clean, it is ready.
7. Remove from the oven, prick a few holes in the top of the cake, then drizzle over the syrup.

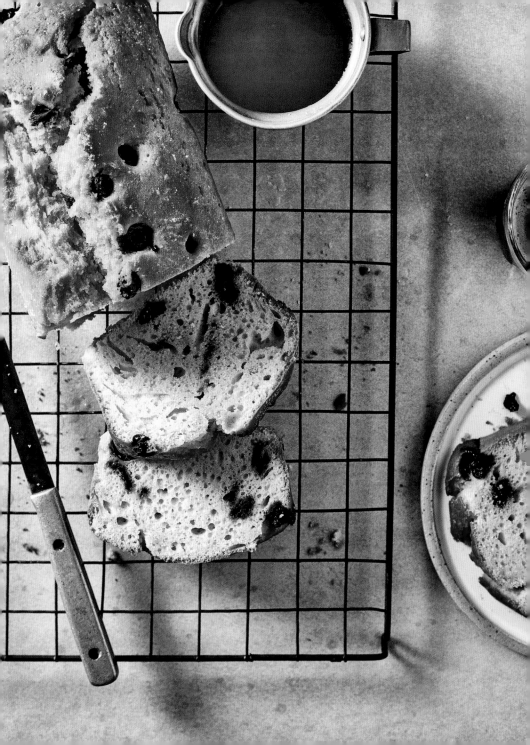

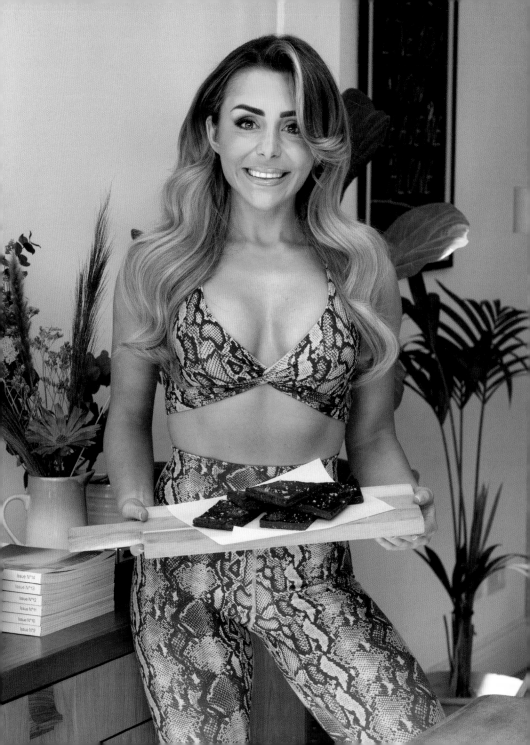

No-bake Protein Chocolate Brownies

If you love a gooey brownie – you're in for a treat. These take next to no time to prepare and require no cooking whatsoever. Just a few hours in the freezer to chill and you're ready to go.

MAKES 10

150g pitted dates
150g whole almonds
90g cocoa powder
60g vanilla protein powder
3 tbsp honey
45g almond butter
2 bananas

1. Blitz the dates, almonds and one-third of the cocoa powder in a food processor until it becomes a fine crumb. Add 5 tablespoons water and blitz again until combined.
2. Line a 20 × 30cm brownie tin with non-stick baking paper and pour in the crumb mixture, pressing down to form an even base.
3. Add the protein powder to the food processor, along with the remaining cocoa powder, the honey, almond butter and bananas. Blitz until smooth.
4. Pour the mixture on top of the crumb base and smooth over with a knife.
5. Pop the tin in the freezer for 2 hours until the top has set. Cut into portions and enjoy.

Carbs 45g

Calories 287

Fat 9g

Protein 8g

Mini Sticky Toffee Puddings

Possibly the most famous dessert on the Courtney Black App. Simple and delicious!

SERVES 2
1 large free-range egg
35g self-raising flour
½ tsp baking powder
1 tbsp granulated
  sweetener
1 tbsp black treacle
25g low-fat spread
Low-calorie cooking spray
1 tbsp maple syrup
150g low-fat custard

1. Preheat the oven to 190°C/375°F/Gas 5.
2. In a large bowl, mix together the egg, flour, baking powder, sweetener, treacle and low-fat spread.
3. Use an electric hand whisk (or a rotary one) to whisk the mixture until combined, smooth and airy.
4. Grab two small heatproof pots or ramekins, spray four times with the cooking spray and rub around the insides with your finger until well greased.
5. Divide the maple syrup between the two pots, then pour equal amounts of cake mixture into each.
6. Bake in the oven for 20 minutes until risen and cooked through. Leave to cool slightly (this will make it easier to remove the puddings from the pots).
7. Once cooled, go around the edges carefully with a knife, flip over and give them a hard tap. The puddings should slowly come out of their pots.
8. Heat the custard and pour around your puddings. Drizzle with any remaining maple syrup if liked.

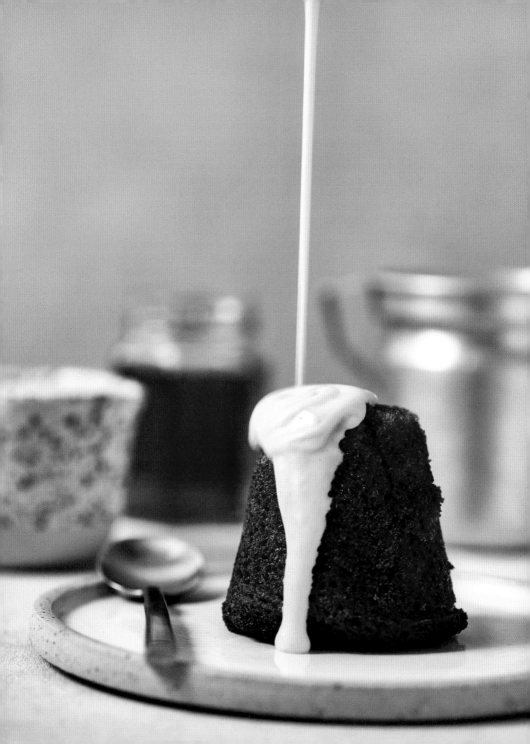

Mini Carrot Cakes

Even though carrot cakes seem healthy, they are usually packed full of sugar and fat. That's exactly why I've developed these low-calorie mini carrot cakes, so you can enjoy the delicious taste without the guilt!

MAKES 10
60g vanilla protein
  powder
150g plain flour
1 tsp baking powder
1 large free-range egg
1 tbsp smooth almond
  butter
1 tbsp maple syrup
180ml semi-skimmed milk
50g apple sauce
50g finely grated carrot
  (reserving a small
  amount for decoration)
1 tsp ground cinnamon

FOR THE FROSTING
150g reduced-fat soft
  cheese
1 tbsp sugar-free maple
  syrup
1 tbsp granulated
  sweetener

1. Preheat the oven to 170°C/325°F/Gas 3.
2. In a large bowl, sift the protein powder, flour and baking powder together and mix until combined.
3. In a separate bowl, whisk the egg and add the almond butter, maple syrup, milk and apple sauce until combined.
4. Add the wet ingredients to the dry and mix until smooth. Stir through the grated carrot and cinnamon.
5. Pour the mixture into the holes of a greased cupcake tin. You should use ten altogether.
6. Bake in the oven for 20 minutes until golden and risen. Remove from the oven and set aside to cool.
7. While cooling, make the frosting: use a spatula to beat the soft cheese, maple syrup and sweetener until light and slightly fluffy. Spoon the mixture over the cooled cakes and top with the reserved finely grated carrot.

Carbs 27.4g

Calories 231

Fat 6.6g

Protein 19.3g

Protein Skillet Blondie

This blonde version of a brownie is sure to satisfy even the most extreme sweet tooth.

SERVES 2

30g plain flour
30g vanilla protein powder
¼ tsp baking powder
1 tbsp granulated sweetener
20ml sugar-free maple syrup
40ml fat-free yoghurt
1 free-range egg
Low-calorie cooking spray
20g chocolate chips
1 scoop low-calorie chocolate ice cream
Sugar-free maple syrup for drizzling

1. Preheat the oven to 170°C/325°F/Gas 3.
2. In a large bowl, sift together the flour, protein powder, baking powder and sweetener.
3. Add the maple syrup, yoghurt and egg and stir until well combined.
4. Lightly grease a small ovenproof frying pan (or cast-iron skillet) with low-calorie cooking spray, then pour in the mixture.
5. Push the chocolate chips down into the mixture and bake on a low rack for 7–9 minutes until set and slightly golden.
6. To serve, add a scoop of chocolate (or your favourite) low-calorie ice cream and an extra drizzle of sugar-free maple syrup.

Carbs 21.8g

Calories 162

Fat 3.3g

Protein 11.8g

White Chocolate and Raspberry Protein Muffins

Satisfy your sweet tooth with these delicious, healthy muffins. Packed with protein, these are the perfect post-workout snack or even a delicious breakfast idea.

MAKES 6

1 banana, mashed
1 free-range egg, beaten
100g fat-free yoghurt
60g vanilla protein powder
20g maple syrup
1 tsp baking powder
1 tsp vanilla extract
100g oats
75ml skimmed milk
24 raspberries
20g white chocolate chips

1. Preheat the oven to 180°C/350°F/Gas 4.
2. In a large bowl, mix together the banana and egg.
3. Add the yoghurt, protein powder, maple syrup, baking powder, vanilla extract and oats. Pour in the milk and mix until combined.
4. Grab a muffin tin and fill with six paper cases. Pour the mixture into the six cases up to halfway. Divide the raspberries between the muffin cases, setting aside six, then divide the white chocolate chips between the muffins, too.
5. Pour the remaining mixture on top of the raspberries and chocolate chips, up to just below the rims of the muffin cases.
6. Top with the remaining raspberries and bake for about 30–35 minutes until golden and cooked through (a wooden skewer inserted into the middle of a muffin should come out clean).

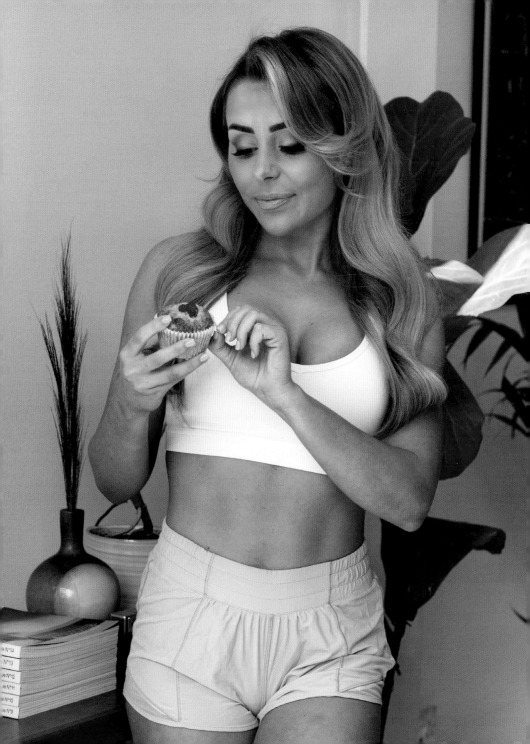

INDEX

ACKNOWLEDGEMENTS

Firstly, I'd like to thank the amazing, hardworking team at HarperCollins Publishers: Helen, James, Georgina, Hattie and Lucy, and also Jenny and Ollie. You really listened to what I wanted for my book and brought the vision to life.

To the shoot team who created the fantastic photos for the book: Anna, Roqa and Jack, thank you for being really accommodating, easy to work with, and for making me feel super comfortable. And Sophie and Pippa for the delicious food photography.

Thanks to Luke, my agent, for being so supportive, believing in me and putting 100 per cent into everything. Thanks to my best friend, Georgia, for always being so supportive.

My mum Colette has been there for me throughout all my struggles. She's worked so hard her whole life, and taught me how to work hard, too. Thanks for everything, Mum.

Finally, thank you so much to all the Instagram community and my followers. I really wouldn't be here if it wasn't for you all!